AF413581

The Art of NATURAL BIRTH

MASTERING SEVEN HABITS FOR A GENTLE ARRIVAL

DR. MEHUL KIRITKUMAR NAYAK

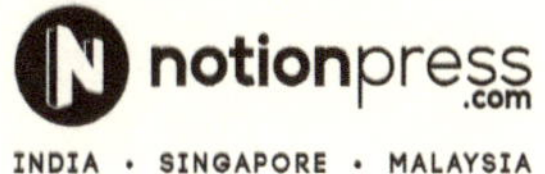

notionpress
.com

INDIA · SINGAPORE · MALAYSIA

Disclaimer

The information presented in **"THE ART OF NATURAL BIRTH"** Mastering Seven Habits for Gentle Arrival is intended solely for educational purposes. This book provides general advice and insights based on research and personal experiences. It is not a substitute for professional medical advice, diagnosis, or treatment.

Consult Your Healthcare Provider

Before making any decisions or changes related to your pregnancy, delivery, or health, it is essential to consult with your healthcare provider. Each pregnancy is unique, and individual medical needs can vary significantly. Only a qualified healthcare professional can provide you with personalized advice and care tailored to your specific situation.

No Guarantees

While this book aims to provide helpful information and tips, it does not guarantee a specific outcome.

Natural delivery depends on numerous factors, many of which are beyond personal control. The methods and habits discussed are meant to support a healthy pregnancy and delivery but do not ensure that a normal delivery will occur.

Potential Concerns

Please be aware that certain practices and habits suggested in this book may not be suitable for everyone. Some recommendations could have potential risks or side e ects depending on individual health conditions and circumstances. Always discuss any concerns or potential risks with your doctor or midwife before implementing any new habits or practices.

Limit of Liability

The author and publisher disclaim any liability for any direct, indirect, incidental, or consequential harm, injury, or damage that may result from the use of the information provided in this book. Readers are responsible for their own health decisions and should act based on the guidance of their healthcare providers.

Acceptance of Terms

By using the information provided in "**THE ART OF NATURAL BIRTH**" **Mastering Seven Habits for Gentle Arrival,** you acknowledge and agree to this disclaimer. If you do not agree to this disclaimer, you should not use or rely on the information in this book.

Contact Information

For any questions or concerns regarding the content of this book, please contact the author or publisher.

Thank you for understanding and respecting the importance of professional medical advice in your pregnancy journey.

Acknowledgement

I'm truly grateful as I look back on the journey of creating this book. I appreciate the universe for giving me this opportunity to share my knowledge. A big thank you goes to all my friends, family, and well-wishers who supported me along the way.

Special thanks to my mother, Manjula Nayak, for the life she has given me, and to my late father, Kiritkumar Nandlal Nayak, whose values guide me every day. My brother Dr Mithilesh is constant moral support for me.My wife Arti, and my children Khushansh and Joyel have been my constant support, filling each day with energy.

I am thankful to Goddess Ichhapuri Mataji for her blessings throughout this project, from the first thought to the final publication.

Dr. Arjunbhai Chaudhary also deserves a heartfelt thanks for his guidance and for providing a platform at Ajooba Hospital that has been crucial in reaching this stage.

My friend and senior Dr Tejasbhai Barot sir has been a pillar of support during every page journey.

Dr. Karsanbhai R Patel also deserves a heartfelt thanks for moral support and offering continuous guidance for developing my personal and professional life.

My friend and mentor, Kunalbhai Mewada, has been a pillar of support. Thanks also to the Arambh musical group for their encouragement, and to A big thank you to my team at Krishna Hospital—Pirabhai Chaudhary, Kishanbhai Chaudhary, Ashokbhai Chaudhary, Prakashbhai Rathod, Gautamben Prajapati, Pravinbhai Thakor, and everyone else there. Your trust in me has been invaluable.

Thank you to Jaya Mirra'ji for skillfully drafting my ideas into this book. Thanks to Dr. Manjunath Sir and the Read for Success community for teaching me that consistency leads to success.I am thankful to all named and unnamed teachers in my life.

Most importantly, I thank every mother who has visited my clinic. Each of you has taught me so much, enriching both my personal and professional life. My deepest gratitude goes out to every mother around the world. Thank you, thank you, thank you for everything.

Contents

Nurturing Habits for a Healthy Pregnancy

*"The journey of a thousand miles
begins with one step."*
– Lao Tzu

What exactly is a habit?

So, what exactly is a habit? Think of it this way: our brains are incredibly smart at saving energy. Just like you might try to save the battery on your phone for it to last longer, your brain does something similar. It looks for ways to do less work on things it does over and over again. And the brain's best trick for this is creating habits.

The beauty of understanding habits as a framework for our lives is that it empowers us to make intentional changes. By identifying the cues that trigger our routines and understanding the rewards we seek, we can begin to craft a life that supports our well-being and aligns with our values, especially during the transformative phase of pregnancy.

How long does it take to form this path, this habit? Well, it's not a one-size-fits-all answer. On average, people say it takes about 66 days, but it can actually take anywhere from 18 to 254 days depending on the person and the habit. You might have heard that it takes 21 days to form a habit, thanks to a surgeon named Maxwell Maltz. He noticed that his patients seemed to get used to their new looks or a missing limb in about three weeks. But the truth is, habits can take much longer to form. It's different for everyone and every habit.

In essence, habits are the invisible architecture of our daily lives. They shape our actions, influence our mood, and ultimately, determine the quality of our lives. During pregnancy, when the well-being of two individuals is interconnected, the significance of cultivating positive habits cannot be overstated. It's a period where the conscious formation of beneficial habits can set the foundation for a healthy and joyful journey into parenthood.

"Motherhood: All love begins and ends there." - Robert Browning

Habits During Pregnancy

Now, why is this especially important during pregnancy? Because pregnancy is a time of big changes, and developing good habits can help you manage these changes better. It's not just about you anymore; it's also about creating the best start for your baby. By understanding how habits work – that they start with a trigger, followed by the behavior, and then a reward that makes you want to do it again – you can start to build habits that will help you through pregnancy and beyond.

- ### *The Habit Loop: A Simple Cycle*

Think of forming a habit as running a loop from a trigger (or cue) to a behavior and then to a reward. This loop is the secret sauce to making any action stick. Here's how it goes: something triggers you to act (that's the cue), you perform the action (that's the behavior), and then you get something good out of it (that's the reward). This reward makes you want to do the behavior again when the same trigger comes up. Over time, this cycle turns the action into a habit.

Pregnancy lasts about 280 days, or roughly 9 months. It's a special time when you might feel more motivated than ever to do what's best for your baby. This period is like a golden window for forming good habits because you have a clear, powerful motivation: the health and well-being of your child.

Working on positive habits consistently during these 280 days can solidify them into long-term patterns. It's a chance to show the world the power of a mother's influence in shaping an advanced, healthy child.

• *The Miraculous Connection*

Here's an amazing fact: during pregnancy, your subconscious mind is linked to your baby's developing mind. The activities you engage in and the habits you form don't just affect you; they help shape your baby's subconscious too. This connection means that the healthy habits you build and the positive environment you create influence your child's development from the very start.

• *Why Develop Habits Now?*

You might wonder, "Can't I just teach my child these habits after they're born?" The thing is, during pregnancy, your baby's brain is like a sponge, absorbing everything. A staggering 80% of a child's brain development happens in the womb. Think of your baby as a blank slate or an empty USB drive at this stage, ready to be filled with valuable data.

Developing good habits now takes advantage of this peak learning time. It's not just about adding knowledge; it's about laying the foundation for your child's entire future. The habits you establish while pregnant can set the tone for the next 99 years of your child's life. A strong, positive start leads to a stronger, healthier future.

So, see these 9 months as your window of opportunity. The habits you form now have the power to benefit your child long before they're born, and well into their future. It's about laying the best possible foundation for them, starting with your actions today.

Let's break down a straightforward approach to forming new habits, especially during pregnancy, using something called the FOGG Behavior Model, often referred to as "Tiny Habits." This method is all about making big changes through small steps.

• *Understanding the FOGG Behavior Model*

At its core, the FOGG Behavior Model simplifies habit formation into three key components: motivation, ability, and triggers. Think of it as a formula:

Behavior = Motivation x Ability x Trigger.

Motivation refers to your desire to do the behavior. It's the reason behind your actions.

Ability is about how easy or hard it is to do the behavior. If something is simpler, you're more likely to do it.

Trigger is the prompt that kicks off the behavior. It's the reminder or the cue to do the habit you're trying to establish.

- ***Tiny Steps Lead to Big Changes***

When it comes to developing new habits during pregnancy, the aim is to start small. Let's use Pranayam (breath control exercises) as an example. Pranayam is great for both you and your baby but might seem daunting at first. So, you start with something simpler: deep breathing ten times. This task is small enough that it doesn't feel overwhelming, making it easier to turn into a habit.

- ***Motivation Matters***

The motivation here is clear: the more oxygen you take in through deep breathing, the more oxygen reaches your baby, promoting their health and reducing the risk of post-birth complications. The thought of giving birth to a healthy and happy baby fuels your motivation to keep up with this practice every day.

Finding the Right Trigger

Next, you tie this new habit of deep breathing to an existing daily routine, like brushing your teeth or taking a shower. This way, every time you finish brushing or showering, it serves as a natural trigger to start your deep breathing exercises. This connection between routine activities and new habits makes the habit stick more effectively.

Types of Triggers

Triggers can come in many forms, and finding the right one can make all the difference:

- **Audio:** The sound of a baby laughing could inspire you to practice your breathing exercises.

- **Visual:** Picturing your future child playing happily can motivate you to stick to your routine.

- **Feeling:** The emotional bond between you and your unborn child can be a powerful trigger.

- **Smell:** A specific scent associated with relaxation could prompt your practice.

- **Environment:** A supportive family environment encourages healthy habits.

- **Time:** Setting a specific time for the activity, like early morning Pranayam, can help cement the routine.

By breaking down the process of habit formation into manageable steps, understanding what drives you, and connecting new habits to your existing routines through effective triggers, you can create lasting changes. This approach is not just about adding beneficial habits during pregnancy but about enhancing your overall lifestyle in a way that's both simple and sustainable.

Habit Formation

In this book, I'm excited to share seven transformative habits that promise not just to smooth the path to a normal delivery but also to encourage comprehensive development in your child. But how can you effectively incorporate these habits into your life? To guide you, I've refined the process into nine practical steps. By applying these steps to the habit of reading books, I'll show you how to seamlessly integrate any habit into your daily routine, enhancing both your life and your child's future.

This process is not just about personal growth; it's about ensuring your well-being and the all-around development of your child during pregnancy.

Step 1: Decide & Write

Start by choosing a goal or quality you want to instill in your child, like courage. Select a book that embodies this trait, such as the life story of Maharana Pratap or Shivaji, and write this decision down. This act of writing solidifies your intention.

Step 2: Understand the Importance

Ask yourself, "Why is this important?" Reading about brave personalities can sow the seeds of courage in your child. Choosing specific books helps nurture specific qualities in your child's development.

Step 3: Identify Your Hot Trigger

Incorporate book reading into an existing part of your routine, like after Pranayam or breakfast. This becomes your hot trigger, a prompt that naturally fits into your day and encourages the new habit.

Step 4: Start with Micro-behaviors

Adopt the FOGG model by starting small. Instead of aiming to read a whole book at once, commit to reading just one page a day. This manageable step can naturally lead to reading more without the pressure.

Step 5: Reward Yourself

Celebrate each reading session with a reward, something you enjoy like a piece of chocolate or a few moments of quiet relaxation. This positive reinforcement makes the habit more appealing.

Step 6: Plan Your Implementation

Set a specific time and place for reading. This structure significantly boosts the likelihood of your habit sticking. Whether it's morning or evening, having a routine creates a natural space for your new habit.

Step 7: Create the Right Environment

Ensure your reading environment is conducive to concentration. Having a designated quiet spot, free from distractions like TV, enhances your focus and enjoyment of reading.

Step 8: Commit for 66 Days

Pledge to read for 30 minutes daily for the next 66 days. This commitment to yourself and your unborn child establishes a powerful motivation to maintain your habit.

Step 9: Find an Accountable Partner

Use habit-tracking apps or join a pregnancy program to share your progress. Having someone to share your

journey which can provide extra motivation and accountability.

Remember, forming new habits can be challenging at first. The initial 20 days might feel tough, but the next 20 days can be a bit easier, and the final stretch becomes enjoyable and rewarding. This process is a testament to the saying,

*"Everything is difficult at the beginning,
messy in the middle, and beautiful in the end."*

As you embark on this journey of habit formation, not only are you preparing yourself for a normal delivery, but you're also laying a strong foundation for your child's future. The habits you develop during pregnancy can have a lasting impact, ensuring you and your child experience the profound benefits of your efforts.

Action Item

Begin a daily gratitude journal. Each day, write down three things you are grateful for in your pregnancy journey. This will help you maintain a positive outlook and appreciate the small joys of this special time.

Chapter 1

"Nurturing Positivity: The Power of a Positive Mental Attitude in Pregnancy"

Positive Mental Attitude

Diving into the concept of Positive Mental Attitude (PMA), we spotlight this habit first for a good reason. PMA acts as a key that unlocks the door to cultivating various beneficial habits, keeping our minds and bodies filled with joy.

PMA might sound new or abstract to some, but it's a principle deeply rooted in the wisdom passed down through generations. It's the age-old advice given to pregnant women to harbor good thoughts, to steer clear of negativity, and to accept positivity in all aspects of life. This is not folklore; it's a practice that has supported the well-being of mothers and their babies for centuries.

To bring this concept to life, let me share a story about two friends, Chingu and Mangu, who were set to take a verbal examination. Both had prepared well and set off for their exam, basking in the beautiful morning sun and enjoying the cool breeze on their bike ride. At a stop, a pigeon overhead dropped its waste, unfortunately hitting both of them. Chingu reacted with anger and frustration, while Mangu remained calm and collected.

Upon reaching the exam, Chingu's frustration spilled over, affecting his performance. He blamed his poor mood on the pigeon incident, letting it overshadow his preparation. Mangu, on the other hand, greeted the examiner with a smile, unaffected by the earlier mishap. He performed well, answering questions with ease and a positive manner. Mangu passed the exam and later shared that he saw the incident as a reminder of how much worse it could have been, jokingly thanking the heavens that elephants don't fly.

This tale highlights the impact our reactions to unforeseen events can have on our outcomes. Pregnancy comes with its set of challenges, such as morning sickness or changes in appetite. Viewing these experiences as part of the incredible journey of bringing a new life into the world can significantly alter your perception and experience of pregnancy.

Adopting a PMA during pregnancy enables you to view these nine months through a lens of gratitude and wonder, recognizing each challenge as part of a larger, beautiful process. This perspective doesn't make the journey more enjoyable; it prepares you to welcome your child with a heart full of positivity.

In essence, PMA teaches us that our outlook can transform our experiences. As you start on the journey of pregnancy, remember the difference in perspective between Chingu and Mangu. This understanding serves as a powerful reminder that the lens through which we view our circumstances can dramatically change our reality.

With this in mind, let's proceed, carrying the wisdom that our attitudes, particularly during significant life moments like pregnancy, can shape not just our own experiences but also the foundational environment for our future children. By cultivating a Positive Mental Attitude, we show the way for a joyful and healthy pregnancy.

Maintaining a positive attitude during challenges can help you navigate the 9 months of pregnancy with ease. If you encounter difficulties, allow me to share an additional story. Would you like to hear it?

This too Shall Pass

Once upon a time, there was a king who had it all: wealth, power, and a kingdom that stretched as far as the eye could see. But, he had a bit of an ego problem, thinking he was invincible because of his riches.

One day, a wise sage visited his court. Seeing the king's arrogance, the sage handed him a note, instructing him to read it when he felt at his highest or his lowest.

Life went on, and the king experienced incredible victories, expanding his kingdom even further. Overwhelmed with joy, he remembered the sage's note. Opening it, he found a simple message: "This too, shall pass." Confused and slightly irritated, he shrugged it off.

However, fortunes change. The king faced a crushing defeat, losing much of what he had. In despair, he opened the note again and read the same message: "This too, shall pass." This time, it struck a chord. He realized that both the good and bad times are temporary. With renewed spirit, he worked hard, rebuilt his kingdom, and regained his glory. But he also learned humility and the importance of a balanced perspective.

So, how does this relate to pregnancy? Well, think of your pregnancy journey as a kingdom of its own. There will be days when you feel on top of the world, glowing and bursting with excitement about the life you're bringing into the world. And there will be days when you're tired, uncomfortable, and maybe even a bit scared about the future.

Just like the king, it's crucial to remember that "This too, shall pass." Embracing a positive mindset isn't about ignoring the tough days; it's about knowing they're just part of the journey. It's understanding that the challenges are temporary and that joy, wonder, and love are on the other side.

A positive mindset during pregnancy helps you navigate the highs and lows with grace. It teaches you resilience, helps you appreciate the good moments even more, and provides strength during the tougher times.

Remember, every kick, every craving, and every moment of restlessness is part of a bigger picture. By maintaining a positive outlook, you're not just caring for yourself but also creating a serene environment for your baby to grow.

Find inspiration in the king's tale and remember: whatever today brings, "This too shall pass." Each moment of your pregnancy journey, whether bright or dark, adds depth and beauty to the story you're weaving with your little one.

The Benefits of Positivity

When you keep a positive mindset during pregnancy, it's like giving yourself and your baby a big, comforting hug. This positive vibe helps you feel calmer and more at peace, making the whole pregnancy experience smoother for you. Think of it as reducing the noise of stress and worry, which allows you to focus on the joy of expecting your little one. This calmness is good for your health and helps you tackle the changes your body is going through with more grace and less discomfort.

For moms-to-be, this positive outlook can lead to better nights of sleep, because you're not tossing and turning with anxiety. You also find yourself with more energy during the day. It's as if your body is saying thank you for keeping things light and hopeful, allowing you to enjoy the pregnancy journey more fully.

And for the babies, the benefits of your positivity are incredibly special. It's like they can feel your happiness and calm from the inside, helping them grow in a cozy and reassuring environment. This can contribute to them being born at a healthy weight, which is a great start to life. Plus, these babies often have a stronger ability to handle stress from a young age. It's like your positive outlook during pregnancy gives them a set of tools for life, helping them face challenges with more resilience. And when it comes to learning and developing, children born to optimistic moms tend to hit their milestones in stride, possibly because they've been nurtured in an environment that encourages growth and happiness.

Maintaining a positive mindset throughout pregnancy doesn't mean overlooking tough days or downplaying the rollercoaster of emotions that may come with this journey. It's completely natural to experience a spectrum of feelings, from overwhelming joy to significant anxiety. The essence of a positive mindset lies in your response to these moments; it's about giving yourself the grace to feel what you're feeling, while also keeping an eye on the broader, beautiful journey you're undertaking.

Acknowledging the hard days doesn't detract from your strength or resilience; it enhances it. When you allow yourself to recognize and move through these feelings, you're practicing a form of self-care that's invaluable, both for you and your baby. It's about finding balance, seeking support when needed, and focusing on the joy and anticipation of meeting your new baby.

A positive mindset during pregnancy is less about constant happiness and more about cultivating an environment of wellbeing and love. It involves practical steps like surrounding yourself with supportive people, engaging in activities that bring you joy, and taking care of your health.

This approach not only benefits you but also creates a peaceful, loving environment for your baby to grow in. Research supports the idea that a calm and positive prenatal environment can have long-term benefits for a child, influencing everything from their physical health to their emotional resilience.

So, while it's okay to not always feel like a beacon of positivity, the effort to return to a hopeful perspective is what counts. This doesn't mean ignoring the realities of pregnancy, but rather choosing to focus on the positives amidst the challenges. It's about preparing yourself and your baby for a future filled with love, happiness, and health. By cultivating a positive mindset, you are establishing the emotional and psychological foundation for your child's life journey. This nurturing process begins even before birth, conveying the powerful message that challenges can be approached with grace, resilience, and an optimistic outlook. It sets the stage for your child to embrace life with confidence and a belief in their ability to overcome obstacles with a positive attitude.

Overcoming Negativity

Think of positivity and negativity as two sides of the same coin. It's pretty rare for them to show up at the same time. The thing is, our brains are wired in a way that most of the time, like 90%, we're leaning towards negative thoughts. This kind of thinking often leads to stress.This tendency towards negative thinking doesn't just color our mood; it can lead to stress, affecting our overall well-being.

Now, the idea of positivity versus negativity isn't about denying the presence of challenges or pretending everything is perfect. It's more about how we choose to respond to the ups and downs of life. Just like you need to recharge your phone's battery after it runs out, our mental and emotional batteries need recharging too. But unlike our phones that passively wait for us to plug them in, recharging our mental state requires active effort.

Staying healthy and positive is similar to taking care of a plant. Neglect it, and it will fade; nurture it, and it thrives. Our minds work similarly. Left unattended, they can drift towards negativity and despair. However, by consciously deciding to focus on positive actions—like exercising, eating well, or engaging in activities that bring joy—we can foster a healthier, more positive outlook.

So, it's crucial to recognize that moving away from stress and towards a more positive frame of mind isn't a passive process. It involves making deliberate choices and taking action towards our well-being. This doesn't mean ignoring the negative but rather acknowledging it and then consciously deciding to focus on the positive, much like choosing to water a plant to ensure its growth despite the dryness around it.

Stress isn't just a fleeting emotion; it can have tangible, long-lasting effects. Research shows that conditions like diabetes, high blood pressure, and other early-onset diseases can trace their origins back to the womb. This concept, known as Fetal Origin of Adult Disease (FOAD), highlights the profound influence of prenatal conditions on a child's long-term health.

The idea here is simple yet significant: the environment we create for our babies before they're even born can set the stage for their future health. This means that a healthy and stress-free pregnancy isn't just beneficial for expectant mothers; it's crucial for the next generation's well-being. Stress during pregnancy doesn't only affect your peace of mind; it can predispose your child to health issues later in life.

Let me tell you a story to explain why fear can be so dangerous and harmful.

Fear has a bigger impact than just dealing with a bad outcome or situation.

In a small village, there lived a sage deeply devoted to his worship in the village temple. The villagers respected his faith and dedication. One day, the God of Death, known as Yamraj, made his way into the village. The sage, upon learning of his arrival, confronted him, curious about his purpose. Yamraj explained that it was time for several villagers to pass away as their time had come, a natural cycle of life and death.

The sage, troubled by this, pleaded with Yamraj not to take anyone from the village. After some discussion, Yamraj, though irritated by the plea, agreed to a compromise. He would only take five people, no more. The sage reluctantly allowed him to proceed under this condition.

As agreed, Yamraj took the lives of five individuals, each due to different causes. When Yamraj reported back to the sage, claiming to have adhered to their agreement, the sage confronted him with the fact that 30 villagers had died, not just five. Yamraj, feeling mocked and considering punishment for the sage, was suddenly faced with the arrival of Narada, a celestial sage.

Narada asked Yamraj to address the sage's concern. Yamraj then clarified, "I only claimed five lives as per our agreement. The additional 25 were taken by their own fear."

Practical tips for maintaining positivity.

During the coronavirus crisis, we noticed that fear played a big role in how people reacted. Sometimes, it's not just the situation itself that's the problem; it's the fear we build around it. Fear can make things seem worse than they are, so it's important to manage it, especially for expectant mothers concerned about their and their baby's well-being.

Let's talk about a powerful tool to combat this fear: meditation. Spending just 30 minutes a day meditating can significantly benefit both you and your baby. Meditation brings a sense of calm and can lead to new achievements in life by providing peace of mind.

The beauty of meditation is that it brings you into the present moment. The mind often dwells on the past or worries about the future, but meditation centers you in the now, where peace resides. This helps to release worries and fosters a sense of tranquility.

Meditation comes in various forms, and it's not just about sitting quietly in a specific posture. Here are three types of meditation that can fit into your daily life:

- **Static Meditation:** This involves finding a quiet space deliberately to focus your mind and calm your thoughts.

- **Active Meditation:** You can practice this during your daily tasks by engaging fully and joyfully in whatever you're doing, giving it your all.

- **Dynamic Meditation:** This is about being completely present in the moment, like when you're dancing or singing.

Incorporating meditation into your routine can be a powerful way to reduce stress and fear, creating a healthier environment for both you and your baby.

"A baby is something you carry inside you for nine months, in your arms for three years, and in your heart until the day you die."
– Mary Mason

Action Item

Practice daily affirmations. Write down five positive affirmations about yourself and your pregnancy, and read them aloud every morning.

Chapter 2

"Nurturing Hope: Setting Achievable Goals in Pregnancy"

Goals Within Reach: Your Pregnancy Journey

"No goal is bigger than courage. It's those who haven't put up a fight that ends up losing. If you don't reach your goal, switch things up, just like trees change their leaves but not their roots."

Setting goals is like drawing a map for a journey you're about to take. It helps you visualize your destination and the path you'll take to get there. In the context of pregnancy, setting goals is all about envisioning the pregnancy experience you hope for and the arrival of a healthy, happy baby.

Goals give you something to aim for. They're like markers along the road, letting you know you're heading in the right direction. When you set a goal, you're saying, *"This is where I want to go, and here's how I plan to get there."* But it's also about being flexible. Sometimes, you might find a roadblock on your path or realize there's a better route. That's where the saying "if you haven't tried, you haven't lost yet" comes into play. It's a reminder that the effort you put in is valuable, and it's okay to adjust your plans if you need to. Just like trees that change their leaves with the seasons but keep their roots stable, you can adapt your goals while staying true to your core intentions.

Understanding Goals in Pregnancy

Now, let's talk about goals in pregnancy. These aren't just any goals; they're deeply personal and tied to one of the most significant experiences of your life. Setting goals during pregnancy can cover a wide range of areas—from health and wellness to emotional preparedness and creating a supportive environment for your baby's arrival.

For instance, you might set a goal to maintain a healthy diet and regular exercise, which are crucial for your baby's development and your well-being. Or you might aim to learn as much as you can about childbirth and parenting, preparing yourself mentally and emotionally for the road ahead. These goals aren't just tasks to check off a list; they're steps toward creating the best possible start for your new family.

Setting goals is just the beginning. The real magic happens in the pursuit of these goals. It's about taking small, consistent steps toward what you want, even when it's hard. It's about celebrating your progress and learning from the challenges. And most importantly, it's about keeping your eye on the prize—a healthy pregnancy and a healthy baby.

But what exactly should these goals look like?

They can range from maintaining a balanced diet and regular exercise to ensuring mental and emotional well-being. For instance, you might set a goal to walk for 30 minutes a day or dedicate time each evening to unwind and connect with your baby. These goals don't have to be monumental tasks; even small, consistent actions can lead to significant, positive changes in your pregnancy experience.

As you navigate through your pregnancy, it's natural to encounter hurdles when trying to establish new routines or habits that you haven't faced before. The journey demands that we push forward with strong determination. It's fascinating to think about how everything in our world begins as a thought before manifesting into something tangible.

The dream of having a healthy baby and experiencing a normal delivery begins in your mind but doesn't become real without action.

Holding onto hope and positive expectations is crucial, but these alone won't bridge the gap between dreams and reality. This is where setting clear, concrete goals during your pregnancy becomes vital. Deciding on the kind of environment you want to provide for your child, the health objectives you aim to achieve, and the steps you plan to take to ensure a safe delivery are all goals that require attention and commitment.

Writing down these goals plays a surprisingly powerful role in making them more real to you. It's a physical act that cements your intentions, transforming them from fleeting thoughts into commitments you're more likely to pursue. When you take the time to jot down "I want to ensure a balanced diet for my baby's development" or "I plan to engage in daily gentle exercises for my well-being and my baby's," you're not just making notes. You're laying down a blueprint for the coming months.

But setting these goals is just the beginning. The next step involves revisiting these written commitments regularly, using them as a guide to steer your daily actions and decisions. It's a way of checking in with yourself, reminding you of your priorities and how each choice you make brings you closer to the healthy pregnancy and delivery you're working towards.

Remember, it's okay to adjust your goals as you move forward. Pregnancy is a dynamic experience, and flexibility can be just as important as determination. What matters most is your commitment to creating the best possible start for your child, grounded in actions that support your well-being and that of your baby.

Example

Taking on the journey of pregnancy, you step into a role much like that of a ship's captain. Let's dive deeper into this analogy to understand the weight of your responsibility over the next nine months. Just as a ship's captain is entrusted with a map to navigate from one point to another, you too are given the task of guiding a precious passenger—your unborn child—safely through the journey of pregnancy to the moment of birth.

The captain's role is crucial; with their knowledge and expertise, they steer the ship, ensuring it reaches its destination as planned. This journey is carefully charted out, and each decision the captain makes influences the outcome. Now, imagine if the ship were left without a captain, or worse if the captain were to ignore the map and give incorrect orders. The risks are clear: the ship could lose its way, or fail to reach its destination on time, putting both the vessel and its cargo in jeopardy.

In the context of your pregnancy, you hold the helm. Your actions, choices, and care directly impact the well-being and development of your baby. The "map" in this scenario includes following a healthy diet, seeking regular medical advice from a trusted healthcare provider, and nurturing both your physical and mental health. These are your navigational tools, guiding you through the waters of pregnancy toward a successful and healthy delivery.

Neglecting these responsibilities is akin to a captain ignoring their duties; without the right care and attention, the journey could face unnecessary risks. The "ship"—your pregnancy—relies on your guidance to ensure the "passenger"—your baby— arrives safely and healthily into the world.

As the captain of this journey, embracing your role means making informed decisions, seeking knowledge, and preparing yourself for the challenges ahead. It involves understanding the importance of each choice you make, from what you eat to how you manage stress, and recognizing that these decisions shape the health and future of your child.

Deciding the goal

Understanding the distinction between desires and goals is key when plotting the course of your pregnancy journey. While a desire is more of a wish or a hope, a goal is a specific, targeted outcome you aim to achieve. Saying "I want a healthy child" is a noble desire, but framing it as "I aim for my child to weigh 3 kgs and have 15% hemoglobin at birth" transforms that desire into a tangible goal. Similarly, aspiring for your child to be smart is wonderful, yet setting a specific goal like "my child will learn to play the piano" gives you a clear target to work towards.

This concept was vividly illustrated by a survey conducted at Harvard University in 1980. When students were asked about their goals and whether they had documented them, the findings were quite revealing. Only 3% had taken the step to write down their goals along with plans to achieve them, 13% had goals but hadn't written them down, and a staggering 84% had no goals at all. Fast forward, and the 3% with clear, written goals and plans were achieving ten times more than their peers. Even the 13% with unwritten goals were outperforming those without any goals.

These insights are incredibly relevant to your pregnancy. They suggest that by simply defining your goals for your pregnancy and your baby's health in clear, written terms, you can significantly enhance your chances of realizing them. This act of writing doesn't just clarify your intentions; it embeds them deeper into your consciousness, setting the stage for action and commitment.

So, how do you apply this to your pregnancy? Begin by reflecting on what specific outcomes you hope for regarding your health and your baby's development. Instead of vague desires, pinpoint measurable targets. Do you wish to maintain a certain level of physical activity? Are there specific nutritional milestones you aim to hit for both your health and the baby's? Writing these goals down acts as a commitment, a roadmap guiding each choice and action you take during these crucial nine months.

But setting the goal is just the start. The next step is crafting a plan to achieve these objectives. What steps will you take to ensure you're getting the necessary nutrients? How will you integrate exercise into your daily routine? Who are the healthcare professionals you'll work with to monitor your progress and your baby's development?

In essence, your written goals for your pregnancy are much more than words on a page. They are commitments to yourself and your future child. By clearly defining these goals and outlining the steps to achieve them, you're not just hoping for a healthy pregnancy and baby; you're actively working towards making it a reality.

The Right Fit

When you're on the search for the perfect healthcare provider for your pregnancy, diving deep into what truly matters to you is essential. Think about what you envision for your childbirth experience. Are you leaning towards a natural birth? Do you prioritize a healthcare provider who takes a more holistic approach to care, or is someone who has a sterling record of managing complex pregnancies and deliveries more up your alley? Initiating your search with these questions can guide you toward a provider whose expertise and values mirror your own.

Digging into a potential doctor's background is more than a checkbox task; it's about finding a match for your specific needs and preferences. Look into their certifications, areas of specialization, and the experiences of other mothers under their care. This can offer invaluable insights into whether they're the right fit for you.

Communication style, however, is where things get truly personal. During pregnancy, you're navigating a landscape filled with both excitement and uncertainty. You need a doctor who doesn't just talk but truly communicates—someone who listens to your concerns, provides clear and compassionate explanations and respects your preferences and decisions. This two-way street of communication can significantly impact your comfort and confidence throughout your pregnancy.

But there's also the practical side of things to consider, like the doctor's availability. It's crucial to have a healthcare provider who has the time to give you the personalized care and attention you deserve. An overbooked doctor might rush appointments or be hard to reach when you have concerns. This is where smaller practices or doctors known for taking a more personalized approach might offer an advantage over those in high-demand or large practices.

Ultimately, finding the right healthcare provider is about aligning your needs and values with their expertise and approach to care. It's a partnership—one that's built on mutual respect, communication, and a shared goal of ensuring a healthy and fulfilling pregnancy and delivery experience.

Questions to Ask

To truly gauge if a doctor is the right match for you, here are some crucial questions you might consider asking:

What is your philosophy on pregnancy and delivery? This question helps you understand their general approach and whether it aligns with your hopes for a normal delivery.

How do you handle complications during pregnancy and labor? While the goal is a smooth, normal delivery, it's important to know how potential challenges would be managed.

Can you tell me about your experience with natural childbirth, if that's your preference? If you're aiming for minimal intervention, knowing their comfort level and success rate with this approach to is key.

What's your stance on pain relief during labor? Understanding their views on options like epidurals or natural pain management techniques can help you decide if their approach matches your own.

How do you support the mother's role in decision-making throughout pregnancy and delivery? This question ensures that your voice will be heard and valued in your care.

Choosing the right doctor is a significant step in your pregnancy journey. It's about more than just expertise; it's about finding someone who shares your values and vision for childbirth. With the right support, you can navigate the path to a healthy pregnancy and delivery with confidence, knowing you and your baby are in good hands.

The Vision of Pregnancy

Following the journey of selecting the right healthcare provider, the next step in preparing for your pregnancy involves crafting a clear vision of what you hope this experience will be like. This vision can serve as a guiding light, helping you navigate through the months ahead with a sense of purpose and clarity.

• *Envisioning Your Ideal Pregnancy*

Visualizing your ideal pregnancy involves more than just daydreaming about the perfect outcome. It's a powerful technique that can positively influence your mindset and emotional well-being. Start by setting aside quiet time to focus on what a healthy pregnancy and normal delivery look like for you. Picture the stages of your pregnancy, from the early signs of growth to the moment you first hold your baby. Think about how you want to feel during this time, the activities you wish to pursue, and the support system you hope to have around you. This mental imagery can reinforce your goals and desires, making them feel more attainable.

• *Milestones and Markers*

To bring your vision into reality, it's helpful to break down your pregnancy journey into specific, measurable goals for each trimester. These milestones serve as checkpoints, ensuring you're on track toward achieving your ideal pregnancy and delivery.

In the first trimester, your goals might include establishing a healthy eating plan, starting a gentle exercise routine, and building a strong relationship with your healthcare provider. These early steps lay the foundation for a healthy pregnancy journey.

Moving into the second trimester, your focus might shift to more detailed planning. This could involve educating yourself on childbirth, exploring prenatal classes, and beginning to prepare your home and life for the arrival of your new family member.

As you enter the final stretch in the third trimester, your goals may center around finalizing your birth plan, ensuring all necessary preparations are in place, and focusing on relaxation and mental preparation for delivery.

Setting these trimester-specific goals provides a clear path forward, helping you make incremental progress toward your vision of a healthy pregnancy and normal delivery. Remember, these milestones aren't just tasks to be checked off; they're steps in the journey of bringing a new life into the world, each contributing to the overall experience you've envisioned.

In essence, visualizing your ideal pregnancy and establishing clear milestones are about more than just planning; they're about creating a positive, healthy environment for both you and your baby. By focusing on what you want to achieve and setting realistic goals to get there, you're taking proactive steps to make your vision of pregnancy a reality.

Overcoming Obstacles

After setting a clear vision for your pregnancy and mapping out key milestones, the next crucial step is preparing for and overcoming any obstacles that might arise. Recognizing potential challenges early on can equip you to navigate them more effectively, ensuring you stay on track toward your goal of a healthy pregnancy and delivery.

Anticipating Challenges

Every pregnancy journey is unique, but there are common hurdles many expectant mothers face. These can range from physical issues like morning sickness or back pain to emotional and mental health challenges such as anxiety or depression. External factors, including access to quality healthcare or support from family and friends, can also play significant roles in shaping your experience.

Identifying these potential obstacles early allows you to seek out resources, advice, and support proactively, rather than reacting to problems as they occur. This foresight can make a considerable difference in how you manage these challenges, reducing their impact on your overall pregnancy experience.

Strategies for Success

Successfully navigating the hurdles of pregnancy involves a combination of practical tools and techniques. Here are some strategies to consider:

- **Build a Support Network:** Surround yourself with people who uplift and support you—family, friends, healthcare providers, or pregnancy support groups. This network can offer practical help, advice, and emotional support when you face challenges.

- **Stay Informed:** Knowledge is power. Educate yourself about the common challenges of pregnancy and childbirth. Understanding what's normal and when to seek help can make you feel more in control and less anxious.

- **Prioritize Self-Care:** Taking care of your physical and emotional well-being is crucial. This includes following a healthy diet, staying active, getting enough rest, and practicing stress-reduction techniques like meditation or prenatal yoga.

- **Prepare for Flexibility:** While having a birth plan is important, be prepared to adapt as needed.

Understanding that some aspects of pregnancy and delivery may not go as planned can help you stay resilient and reduce disappointment.

- **Communicate Openly with Your Healthcare Provider:** Keep the lines of communication open with your doctor or midwife. Discuss any concerns or symptoms you're experiencing, no matter how small they seem. This ensures you receive the right care at the right time.

- **Focus on What You Can Control:** Concentrate your energy on aspects of your pregnancy journey that are within your control, such as attending prenatal appointments, eating well, and preparing your home and family for the new arrival.

- **Practice Positive Visualization:** Regularly visualize successful outcomes for any challenges you might face. This positive mental rehearsal can boost your confidence and help you approach hurdles with a problem-solving mindset.

Overcoming obstacles during pregnancy isn't about avoiding problems altogether but about equipping yourself with the knowledge, resources, and support to manage them effectively. By anticipating potential challenges and adopting these strategies, you can maintain your focus on your goals, adapt as necessary, and navigate your pregnancy journey with confidence and grace.

"A mother's joy knows no bounds when she brings forth a new life into this world. It is an experience beyond compare."
– Unknown

Action Item

Create a vision board for your pregnancy goals. Include images and words that inspire you and represent your hopes and dreams for your pregnancy and birth experience.

Chapter 3

"Nurturing Every Moment: Embracing Daily Routines in Pregnancy"

"The moment a child is born, the mother is also born. She never existed before. The woman existed, but the mother, never. A mother is something absolutely new."
– Rajneesh

Daily Routine

A routine is a collection of habits or tasks you do often, creating a steady flow for your day. It's like putting together pieces of a puzzle to build a clear picture of how your day looks, giving you a plan to follow. This planning can be beneficial, especially when you're pregnant and going through a lot of changes.

Having a routine means you're doing certain things at about the same time each day. This could be eating meals, exercising, working, resting, or any other activity important to your health and well-being. It's a way to ensure you're taking care of yourself by setting aside time for everything you need to do, including taking a break when needed.

Why is a routine so important for a normal pregnancy? Well, it brings a sense of stability and balance to what can be an unpredictable time. Your body is going through incredible changes, and your emotions might be on a rollercoaster ride. A daily routine can act as an anchor, helping you focus on what's important and keeping you grounded.

Here's what a supportive daily routine can offer:

- **Nutrition:** Regular meal times ensure you're fueling your body and your baby with the right nutrients at the right intervals.

- **Exercise:** Incorporating light exercise into your routine can enhance your physical well-being and mood, as well as prepare your body for childbirth.

- **Rest:** Pregnancy can be tiring. A routine helps you make sure you're getting enough rest, with regular sleep times and opportunities for daytime relaxation.

- **Hydration:** Setting reminders to drink water throughout the day is crucial for maintaining the amniotic fluid levels and supporting your increased blood volume.

- **Stress Management:** Dedicating time to activities that reduce stress, such as prenatal yoga, meditation, or simply reading a book, can significantly impact your emotional health.

Having a routine doesn't mean scheduling every minute of your day. It's about having a basic plan to guide you through the day, helping you feel more in control and less stressed by making sure you don't forget important things in daily life.

What's an Ideal Routine?

Talking about an ideal daily routine, it's a set of activities that help make us better when we do them every day. Think of "din" meaning day and "charya" meaning behavior. A routine is like a good plan for the day that helps us do things the way nature does, in a nice, orderly way. This plan isn't just for doing things; it's also about making our minds and bodies strong and helping us fight off sickness.

Key Parts of a Good Daily Plan

- **Doing Things Regularly:** It's all about doing certain things at the same time every day. This helps our bodies and minds get used to a pattern, making us feel better and keeping us healthy.

- **Making a Plan:** A good routine is more than just doing things whenever; it's about having a plan. This might mean deciding when you'll eat, work, move your body, chill out, or sleep. It makes sure every part of your day is helping you stay healthy.

- **Keeping Things Balanced:** It's important to do different kinds of activities that make you feel good in all ways—mentally, in your heart, in your body, in your feelings, and with friends or family. Keeping a balance means you're taking care of every part of yourself.

- **Making a Big Difference:** Following a routine doesn't just help day-to-day; it can actually do big things for our health over time. Scientists say that doing the same healthy things regularly can even make our genes work better, helping us live longer and healthier.

How to Create Your Ideal Routine

Making a daily routine that's just right for you means more than just sticking to a schedule. It's about living in a way that's in sync with how nature works, taking care of what your body and mind naturally need. This kind of harmony isn't just good for you; it makes everything around you better—making the world a happier place because you're feeling good and doing well.

By sticking to a well-thought-out plan every day, we're not only making sure we're living healthier but also making life more enjoyable and meaningful in many ways.

Understanding how powerful a daily routine can show us that our every day habits can truly shape our lives for the better. By planning our days carefully and sticking to routines that take care of our whole selves, we're opening the door to a life filled with health, happiness, and peace.

Epigenetic effect

Exploring the fascinating world of epigenetics, we delve into how our genes, those tiny blueprints we inherit from our parents and ancestors, can be influenced not just by their original structure but by our lifestyle and environment. This field of study shines a light on how our daily habits and the world around us can directly impact our genetic expression.

Understanding Epigenetics

At its core, epigenetics involves changes in how our genes work. Interestingly, these changes don't alter the DNA sequence itself but affect how genes are turned on or off. Think of it as having a sophisticated control system for your genes, akin to updating the software on your computer without changing the hardware. This system ensures that genes necessary for certain bodily functions are active when needed, while others remain dormant.

The Origins of Our Genes

Our genes are inherited from both parents, carrying the legacy of our ancestors within us. This genetic inheritance is the foundation of our biological makeup, determining everything from our eye color to our susceptibility to certain health conditions. However, epigenetics introduces the concept that the expression of these genes can be modified by our actions and environment.

The Influence of Daily Rhythms on Genetics

Our bodies are governed by a natural time-keeping system known as the circadian cycle, or biological clock, which orchestrates the activities of our entire body. This cycle has the remarkable ability to activate or deactivate thousands of genes, influencing various bodily functions. Disruptions in our routine—such as irregular eating or sleeping patterns—can confuse this biological clock, leading to miscommunication with our genes. This misalignment can affect our sleep patterns, hormonal balance, digestion, metabolism, and even cardiovascular health.

The concept of epigenetics was introduced by Conrad Hal Waddington in 1942, emphasizing the intricate relationship between our genes and the environment. His insights laid the groundwork for understanding how external factors like diet, stress, and exposure to toxins can influence gene expression, potentially impacting our health and well-being.

Practical Implications

This connection between our lifestyle and genetic expression highlights the importance of maintaining a balanced daily routine. By aligning our habits with our body's natural rhythms—ensuring regular sleep, balanced nutrition, and consistent physical activity—we can support optimal gene expression. This not only enhances our immediate physical and mental health but may also have long-term implications for our genetic legacy.

In essence, the dynamic field of epigenetics offers a powerful reminder of our own role in shaping our health and destiny. By making conscious choices about how we live our lives, we can positively influence the way our genes express themselves, paving the way for better health, not just for ourselves but for future generations.

Circle of A Day

Diving into a day in the life of a pregnant woman, it's helpful to think of the daily routine as divided into four main parts: morning, afternoon, evening, and night. Each part of the day has its own set of activities that, when put together, support a healthy pregnancy.

the ideal morning routine for a pregnant woman, focusing on activities that nurture both body and mind, enhancing overall well-being.

Morning Routine for a Healthy Pregnancy

- **Morning Awakening (Brahma Muhurta):** Waking up during Brahma Muhurta, which is considered an ocean of positive energy, is highly recommended. This time, just before dawn, is believed to be perfect for spiritual activities. Engaging in asana, pranayama, chanting, and meditation can significantly increase and stabilise your life force energy. It's a peaceful time when the environment is calm, your mind is most alert, and self-awareness is heightened, making it ideal for connecting with universal energy. Scientific studies, including those by Pierce J. Harvard and Dr. Michael Roizen, have shown that this time of day is characterized by alpha waves in the brain, which are associated with relaxation and a state of wakeful rest. This is also when serotonin, a mood-enhancing hormone, is released, boosting positivity and concentration. Moreover, the prevalence of negative ions in the air during this time can increase oxygen flow to the brain, leading to greater alertness and mental energy.

- **Usha Paan (Early Morning Water Therapy):** Drinking 2-3 glasses of lukewarm water early in the morning, preferably in a squatting position, helps remove toxins from the body. This practice cleanses the kidneys, intestines, and skin, leading to better organ health and activity. It also aids in preventing and addressing digestive issues like gas and acidity, boosts immunity by diluting and washing away the bacteria that multiply in the mouth overnight, and contributes to the development of kinesthetic intelligence.

- **Micro Breakfast:** A small breakfast consisting of almonds, dates, walnuts, and sattu provides a nutritious start to the day. These foods offer essential vitamins, minerals, and fiber, supporting physical health and mental clarity.

- **Household Chores with Music:** Incorporating music into daily activities can significantly reduce fatigue and make routine tasks more enjoyable. Whether it's classical or rock music, the right tunes can stimulate the brain in positive ways, enhancing mental and emotional well-being.

Research supports the idea that children benefit from exposure to good sound, suggesting that melodious music can increase the productivity of brain neurons.

- **Yogasana with Music:** Combining yoga with soothing music helps in calming the mind, improving balance, and enhancing concentration.

- **Pranayama (Breath Control):** Practices like Anulom-Vilom and Bhramari help distribute life force throughout the lungs, nervous system, and brain, supporting spiritual growth and expanding personal energy.

- **Meditation and Chanting:** Engaging in meditation and chanting can have profound effects on the brain, similar to tuning into specific radio frequencies. This practice helps focus the senses, strengthen decision-making abilities, and enhance learning and awareness.

The Science Behind the Routine

Chanting mantras like the Gayatri Mantra can have positive effects on the brain. Research by Dr. Howards Steingeril from Hamburg University in America found that the Gayatri Mantra produces 110,000 sound waves per second, making it one of the most powerful hymns globally. Neuroscientist James Hartzell from Spain observed improvements in cognitive function with the Sanskrit effect. Dr. Rama Jaya Sundar from AIIMS in Delhi, India also studied the effects of the Gayatri mantra. According to Arthur Koestler, "Gayatri Mantra has the power of a thousand atomic bombs".

Breakfast Choices

By adopting this structured morning routine, pregnant women can significantly enhance their physical, mental, and spiritual health, setting a positive tone for the rest of the day.

For breakfast, a nutritious mix can set the day off right, especially during pregnancy. Here's a simple yet powerful breakfast idea:

- **Fenugreek Seeds:** Just 5 grams. They're good for boosting your immunity and helping with any inflammation.

- **Moong (Green Grams):** About 25 grams. These are great for digestion and also pack a punch with vitamins and minerals.

- **Celery:** Just a bit of it. It's not only refreshing but also helps with digestion and can calm any stomach issues like gas or bloating.

- **Gram (Chickpeas):** 15 grams of it. Chickpeas are full of fiber which keeps your digestive system running smoothly.

- **Black Salt:** Add according to your taste. It adds not just flavor but also aids in digestion.

- **Peanuts:** 10 grams. They're a good source of protein and also help with feeling full.

This breakfast is packed with vitamins that boost your immune system and minerals that are essential for the development of bones, teeth, heart, muscles, and nerves in both you and your baby. The fiber in this meal helps prevent constipation, a common issue during pregnancy. The enzymes, particularly from celery, aid in better digestion and nutrient absorption, while the antioxidants from sprouts add an extra layer of health benefits.

Afternoon Routine for a Healthy Pregnancy

Incorporating soothing music into your day as you engage in household activities can transform routine tasks into moments of joy and relaxation. Whether you're preparing food, tidying up, or engaging in any other daily chore, the backdrop of calming tunes can uplift your spirits.

Preparing Food with Awareness

When making meals, think of it as nurturing not just the body but also the mind and spirit. The process of cooking can be a way to express creativity and care.

Aim for Satvik food—vegetarian dishes that are fresh, easy to digest, and packed with nutrients like vitamins, minerals, fiber, and antioxidants. While cooking, maintaining positive thoughts can infuse the food with good energy, echoing the concept of Baliveshva Yagya, where the food is seen as an offering made with the fruits of honest labor. Strive for a balanced diet where your meal includes a good mix of proteins, carbohydrates, fats, and vitamins, following a 4:4:1:1 ratio for well-rounded nourishment.

Remember, it's best to eat fruits a few hours after meals to optimize digestion. Practicing Vajrasana, a simple yoga pose, post-meal can aid in this process by facilitating the release of digestive hormones and directing blood flow to aid in digestion.

Rest and Engagement

After lunch, dedicating time to rest and engage in leisure activities can significantly contribute to your well-being:

- **Rest:** Aim for a brief nap of about half an hour to rejuvenate your body and mind.

- **Stories and Satsang:** Spend another half hour listening to stories or engaging in meaningful conversations. This can be a powerful way to connect with your culture, values, and spiritual beliefs.

- **Hobbies:** Dedicate about an hour to hobbies that stimulate your mind and creativity. Puzzles, chess, and Sudoku challenge your logical thinking; arts and crafts enhance your fine motor skills as well as your visual and spatial understanding. Activities like writing in a journal or essays sharpen your linguistic and intrapersonal skills while spending time with children and elders helps develop interpersonal skills and a deeper connection to the natural world around you.

- **Mindfulness:** Finally, incorporating a session of Dhyan (meditation) into your routine can center your thoughts and emotions, preparing you for the rest of the day with clarity and peace. Follow this with a light snack (Nasta) that aligns with your body's nutritional needs and keeps you energised until dinner.

Incorporating these elements into your daily routine not only boosts your physical health but also nurtures your mental, emotional, and spiritual well-being. This methodical yet adaptable approach to your day helps maintain balance, fulfillment, and harmony within yourself and your environment.

Evening Routine for a Healthy Pregnancy

Spending time with family in the evening can turn into a cherished part of your day, especially with activities like pooja or prayer. This simple tradition is much more than a religious ritual; it's a powerful way to bring everyone closer. Ending each day by gathering with your loved ones, and sharing a quiet moment of gratitude and reflection is a beautiful way to cultivate connection and appreciation. It's about pausing from the rush of life to appreciate what we have and those around us.

In these moments, when you're all together, you can share how your day went, talk about things that made you happy, or even things that didn't go as planned. It's a safe space where everyone can open up, leading to deeper conversations and understanding among family members. This practice becomes a daily reminder of your support for one another, strengthening your bond.

It's a chance for everyone to stop, look around at the faces of family members, and really feel grateful for being together.

Moreover, this evening ritual can be a stress reliever. In a world that's always moving fast, taking this time to slow down and connect on a deeper level can be incredibly calming. It reminds everyone of the bigger picture and the importance of family amidst life's challenges.

Creating such a routine enriches the family's emotional landscape, making each evening a special time of connection and peace. It teaches everyone, especially children, the value of gratitude, the strength found in family, and the beauty of ending the day together on a positive note.

Relaxing with Music

As the evening goes on, it's lovely to bring music into whatever you're doing. Music has a way of making everything feel nicer, whether you're finishing up some chores, preparing dinner, or just sitting and relaxing. You could listen to soft music, sing, or even play music yourself. Music helps calm your mind and can bring out your creative side, making everyday tasks more fun.

Bringing the family together for prayer and enjoying music are simple ways to make the evening peaceful and happy. These activities are not just about ending the day well; they help everyone in the family feel good and grow closer. It shows how little moments and activities can make a big difference in how we feel and connect with our loved ones.

Night Routine for a Healthy Pregnancy

Moving into the night, let's talk about how to wrap up your day in a way that supports both your health and your connection with your family, especially during pregnancy.

Nighttime Routine

- **Light Dinner:** Eating something light for dinner can really help your body digest better and prepare you for a good night's sleep. It means choosing foods that won't make your stomach work too hard.

- **Evening Walk:** Taking a gentle walk with your husband can be a lovely way to spend some quality time together. It's not just good for your physical health but also gives you a chance to talk and bond.

- **Garbh Samvad with Father:** This is a special time when the father-to-be can talk or sing to the baby in the womb. It's a beautiful way to start building a bond between the father and the baby early on.

- **Turmeric Milk:** Drinking milk mixed with a little turmeric and honey is not only tasty but also packed with health benefits. Turmeric has properties that help fight off skin problems, boost your immunity, and even help you sleep better.

The honey adds a touch of sweetness and its own set of benefits.

- **Swadhyaya – Food for the Soul:** Swadhyaya means taking some time to read and reflect on meaningful literature. It could be anything that inspires you or makes you think. This practice sharpens your mind, helps you make better decisions, and cleanses your inner self.

- **Sadhana of Tatvabodh and Day Analysis:** Before the day ends, take a moment to think about all the good things you did and how you can carry those forward. Also, think about any mistakes and how you can avoid them in the future. This is a way to dedicate yourself to continuous improvement and keep your moral compass in check.

- **Review of Ideal Routine Chart:** Finally, take a quick look at your routine chart. See what went well and what didn't. This helps you stay on track with your goals and keep improving your daily routine.

- **Intrapersonal Skills:** This entire process of wrapping up your day with reflection, bonding, and planning for the next day is great for developing intrapersonal skills. It helps you understand yourself better, manage your emotions, and plan for a better tomorrow.

By following these steps, you can end your day on a positive note, ensuring you and your baby are getting the care and attention needed. This routine is not just about ending the day but about enriching your life and the life of your growing family with healthy practices, meaningful connections, and personal growth.

Involving Your Support Network

As you navigate through your pregnancy, involving your support network in your daily routine can significantly enrich your journey. Your partner, family, friends, and even your broader community can play a pivotal role in providing support, love, and care during this special time.

Engaging Your Partner

- **Share Your Routine:** Let your partner know about your daily routine and how they can be a part of it. Whether it's joining you for a night walk, helping with meal preparation, or simply spending quiet time together, sharing these moments can strengthen your bond.

- **Plan Together:** Involve your partner in planning your routine, especially when it involves health check-ups, exercise, or diet plans. This not only makes them feel included but also helps you both stay on the same page regarding your pregnancy journey.

- **Communicate Needs and Expectations:** Openly discussing what you need from your partner and what they can expect from you is crucial. Clear communication can help avoid misunderstandings and ensure both of you are contributing positively to the pregnancy experience.

Involving Your Community

- **Seek Support from Family and Friends:** Don't hesitate to reach out to your family and friends for support. Whether it's needing someone to talk to, help with household chores, or advice on pregnancy, your loved ones can offer invaluable support.

- **Join Pregnancy Groups:** Connecting with other expectant mothers through pregnancy groups or classes can provide a sense of community and shared experience. It's a great way to learn from others, share your own experiences, and make new friends who are going through similar changes.

- **Engage in Community Activities:** Participating in community activities, whether it's a prenatal yoga class, a pregnancy workshop, or a mothers' group, can enhance your social well-being and provide additional support and information.

- **Volunteer for Shared Tasks:** Encourage family members to be involved by assigning tasks that they can take up to support you, like accompanying you to doctor's appointments or setting up the baby's nursery. This not only lightens your load but also helps them feel more connected to the pregnancy.

By actively involving your partner and community in your daily routine, you create a supportive network that not only assists you through the practical aspects of pregnancy but also provides emotional support and companionship. This collective effort can make your pregnancy journey more joyful, less stressful, and deeply enriching for everyone involved.

Adapting Your Routine

As you move through your pregnancy, you'll find your body changing in ways that might surprise you. It's normal and means you might need to switch up how you do things every day. Here's a simpler look at making those changes work for you.

First off, pay attention to what your body's telling you. Some days you'll feel like you can take on the world. Other days, not so much. It's okay to slow down and rest when you need to. This is your body's way of saying it's time to take it easy.

If you used to jog or do high-energy workouts, you might need to find gentler ways to stay active. Walking, prenatal yoga, or swimming are great options that are easier on your body but still keep you moving.

Work might also need a tweak. Sitting at a desk all day or standing for long hours can get tough. It's worth talking to your boss about making your workspace more comfortable, or even adjusting your hours if you're feeling really worn out.

Sleep becomes super important now. You might find yourself needing more sleep than usual, or wanting to nap during the day. Try to make sleep a priority. It might mean turning in earlier or finding a comfy way to prop yourself up in bed.

Eating right is another big one. Your body needs all kinds of nutrients to help your baby grow, but you might also deal with cravings or morning sickness. Try to fill up on foods that are good for you and your baby, even if that means eating smaller, more frequent meals.

Lastly, it's okay to ask for help. Whether it's your partner, a family member, or a friend, let them know what you need. It could be help with shopping, cleaning up, or just having someone to chat with when you're feeling overwhelmed.

Remember, adapting your routine isn't about sticking strictly to do's and don'ts. It's more about finding what works best for you and your baby during this special time. You're learning to flow with the changes, making adjustments as you go.

And if I had to leave you with a thought, it'd be this: *"Pregnancy is a journey of change, not just for your body but for your life. It's about growing, in more ways than one."* So, take each day as it comes, listen to your body, and don't be afraid to do things a bit differently than before.

Action Item

Establish a simple, nurturing morning routine that includes a few minutes of stretching, a healthy breakfast, and a moment of mindfulness or meditation.

Chapter 4

"Nurturing the Soul: Spiritual Practices for a Healthy Pregnancy"

" Faith can move mountains."
(The Bible; paraphrased from
Matthew 21:21)

Spiritual nourishment is about feeding your soul and inner self, just like how you nourish your body with food. It's about finding peace, meaning, and connection beyond the physical aspects of life. During pregnancy, a time of significant change and anticipation, spiritual nourishment takes on a special importance. It's not just about taking care of your body to ensure a healthy pregnancy, but also about caring for your mind and spirit, preparing yourself emotionally and spiritually for the journey of motherhood.

Pregnancy is a unique time for spiritual growth and reflection. It offers an opportunity to connect more deeply with yourself, your baby, and the world around you. Engaging in spiritual practices during this time can provide comfort, strength, and clarity as you navigate the physical and emotional changes of pregnancy. It helps you nurture a sense of peace and strength, creating a positive space for your little one to thrive.

Feeding Your Soul

Feeding your soul, especially during pregnancy, is about turning inward and nurturing your innermost self. It's like watering a plant not just to keep it alive, but to help it thrive and blossom. For a pregnant woman, this involves finding moments and practices that fill her with a sense of serenity, hope, and joy.

When we talk about feeding your soul in pregnancy, it's about engaging in activities and practices that make you feel connected, peaceful, and positive. It could be anything that brings you a sense of calm and happiness—like spending quiet moments in nature, meditating, praying, or simply doing things you love, like reading or listening to music. These practices help you create a strong, nurturing environment for your baby even before they are born.

The idea is to fill your life with moments that uplift you spiritually. This doesn't just benefit you by reducing stress and enhancing your emotional well-being; it also has a positive impact on your baby. When you're in a state of mental and emotional harmony, it contributes to creating a peaceful, loving environment that surrounds your baby as they grow.

Actively searching for and welcoming moments and practices that enrich your inner life, giving you and your baby strength, peace, and joy.

When we delve into the essence of spiritual practices, especially during pregnancy, we're looking at ways to connect with something greater than ourselves—be it through mindfulness, prayer, meditation, or gratitude. These practices offer a bridge to an inner world of peace and understanding, crucial during the transformative journey of pregnancy.

For a pregnant woman, this balance is vital not just for her own well-being but also for the emotional and spiritual development of the baby she carries. Engaging in spiritual practices during pregnancy isn't about adhering to a specific religious belief; rather, it's about fostering a deep sense of connection and tranquility within oneself.

Why It Matters in Pregnancy

During pregnancy, the body undergoes significant changes, which can be both exhilarating and stressful.

Amidst this whirlwind of physical transformations, the mind and spirit can feel unsettled, searching for anchor points. Here, spiritual practices come into play, offering moments of stillness, reflection, and profound connection. They act as gentle reminders of the miracle of life being nurtured within, helping expectant mothers to tune into the rhythms of their bodies and the whispers of their hearts.

The Essence of Spiritual Practices

Mindfulness: This is about being fully present in the moment, aware of your body, your thoughts, and your surroundings, without judgment. For an expectant mother, mindfulness can transform routine pregnancy check-ups and moments of rest into opportunities for deep connection with her baby.

Gratitude: Cultivating a practice of gratitude during pregnancy can shift focus from discomfort and anxiety to appreciation and joy. Simple acts of acknowledging the good in each day can elevate an expectant mother's spirit and foster a positive environment for her baby.

Meditation: Meditation offers a sanctuary of calm amidst the storm of emotions and changes. It can be particularly powerful in strengthening the bond between mother and baby, as the quiet space created during meditation is shared between the two.

Prayer and Reflection: For those inclined, prayer can be a source of strength and comfort, a way to seek blessings and express hopes for the unborn child. Reflection, whether spiritual or personal, allows expectant mothers to explore their fears, dreams, and hopes in a safe, internal space.

Integrating these spiritual practices into daily life during pregnancy doesn't require grand gestures. It's about finding small, manageable moments to pause, breathe, and connect—be it through a few minutes of meditation in the morning, jotting down things you're grateful for at night, or simply being fully present as you prepare for the day.

The Benefits of Spiritual Practices

The benefits of integrating spiritual practices into your pregnancy journey are profound and multifaceted. Engaging in activities such as mindfulness, gratitude, and positive affirmations doesn't just positively influence your emotional state.

Mindfulness

Mindfulness during pregnancy is like tuning into a conversation between your body and your baby, listening closely with kindness and without judgment. It's about noticing the sensations in your body, the rhythm of your breath, and even the tiny movements of your baby as they grow. This level of attention can transform how you experience pregnancy.

How Mindfulness Helps

Stress Reduction: Pregnancy can come with worries and uncertainties. Mindfulness brings your attention to the present, helping to clear the clutter of future anxieties or past regrets. By focusing on the now, such as feeling the sensation of your baby moving or simply being aware of your breathing, you reduce stress levels. Lower stress is beneficial for your health and creates an optimal environment for your baby's development.

Emotional Balance: Mindfulness encourages you to observe your emotions without getting swept away by them. This can be especially useful during pregnancy when emotions can fluctuate widely. Recognizing an emotion, acknowledging it, and letting it pass without harsh judgment can lead to greater emotional stability.

Enhanced Connection with Your Baby: Paying mindful attention to your pregnancy can deepen your bond with your baby before they are born. Simple practices like gently resting your hands on your belly and focusing on the sensation of your baby's kicks or movements foster a sense of closeness and anticipation.

Physical Awareness and Comfort: Being mindful can also increase your awareness of your body's needs. It might prompt you to adjust your posture for comfort, recognize when you need rest, or even identify cravings that signal nutritional needs. This heightened body awareness supports both your well-being and your baby's growth.

Preparation for Labor: Mindfulness practices can equip you with coping skills for labor. Focusing on your breath and staying present can help manage discomfort and make the labor process more manageable.

Incorporating Mindfulness into Pregnancy

Integrating mindfulness into your daily routine can be straightforward. It might involve taking a few minutes each morning to breathe deeply and set intentions for the day, practicing yoga designed for pregnant women, or simply pausing throughout the day to check in with yourself and your baby. These moments of mindfulness strengthen the emotional and spiritual connection between you and your baby, enhancing your pregnancy journey.

Gratitude

Practicing gratitude during pregnancy is like shining a light on the beauty and blessings that surround you, even amidst the challenges and changes. It's about acknowledging the small joys and the immense miracles, cultivating an attitude that cherishes and appreciates the journey of bringing a new life into the world.

Why Gratitude Matters

Shifts Perspective: Pregnancy, while miraculous, can also be fraught with discomforts and worries. Focusing on gratitude helps shift your perspective from what's bothering you or causing fear to what's good and hopeful around you. This shift isn't about ignoring challenges but about balancing them with positive acknowledgments, making the whole experience more rounded and fulfilling.

Boosts Mood: Recognizing and appreciating the good in your life naturally elevates your mood. This uplift in spirits is crucial during pregnancy, a time when hormonal fluctuations can impact emotional well-being. A happier mood not only makes the pregnancy journey more enjoyable for you but also creates a positive environment for your baby to develop.

Reduces Stress: Gratitude has the power to calm the mind and soothe the nerves, effectively reducing stress levels. Stress is not uncommon in pregnancy, but its management is key to both maternal and fetal health. By focusing on gratitude, you engage in natural stress relief that benefits both you and your baby.

Enhances Bonding with Your Baby: When you practice gratitude, you're also more likely to feel grateful for the life growing inside you. This can enhance the emotional bond you feel with your baby even before they are born. Feeling thankful for the kicks, the growth, and even the challenges helps deepen your connection to your pregnancy and your baby.

Practicing Gratitude in Pregnancy

Incorporating gratitude into your daily routine can be simple and requires no special tools:

Gratitude Journal: Keep a notebook where you jot down three things you're grateful for each day. These could be as simple as a sunny morning, a supportive partner, or the feeling of your baby moving.

Gratitude Moments: Throughout your day, pause to acknowledge moments of beauty or kindness. It could be a stranger's smile, a delicious meal, or a quiet moment to yourself.

Gratitude Reflections: Before going to bed, reflect on your day and think about what you were most thankful for. This practice can help end your day on a positive note, contributing to better sleep.

Gratitude Sharing: Share your feelings of gratitude with others, especially with your partner or family. This not only multiplies the joy but also strengthens your relationships during this significant phase of your life.

Positive affirmations

Positive affirmations during pregnancy are like a gentle, reassuring voice within you, offering encouragement and strength as you navigate the journey of bringing a new life into the world. These affirmations are powerful tools for maintaining a positive outlook and fostering an environment of love and confidence, both for yourself and your developing baby.

The Power of Positive Affirmations

Building Confidence: Pregnancy is a profound journey that requires strength and resilience. Affirmations such as "I am strong" or "I trust my body's ability to give birth" reinforce your belief in your own strength and capabilities. This self-belief is crucial as you prepare for childbirth, helping you approach labor with confidence rather than fear.

Reducing Anxiety: It's natural to feel anxious or uncertain about the changes your body is undergoing and the impending responsibilities of motherhood. Positive affirmations can serve as calming reminders of your ability to handle these changes. Phrases like "I am surrounded by love and support" can alleviate feelings of anxiety, making the pregnancy journey more peaceful.

Enhancing Emotional Well-being: Your emotional health during pregnancy is as important as your physical health. Affirmations that focus on positivity, such as "Every day, I feel more connected to my baby," nurture feelings of joy and anticipation. This positive emotional state benefits not only you but also contributes to a nurturing environment for your baby's growth.

Supporting Physical Health: The mind-body connection is powerful, and a positive mindset can have tangible benefits on physical health. Affirmations like "My body is doing a wonderful job growing my baby" can help you tune into and appreciate the incredible work your body is performing. This positive mindset can encourage healthy behaviors, further supporting your physical well-being.

Integrating Positive Affirmations into Pregnancy

Incorporating positive affirmations into your daily routine can be simple and easily adapted to fit your lifestyle:

Morning Affirmations: Start your day by repeating a few chosen affirmations. This sets a positive tone for the day ahead.

Affirmation Reminders: Place sticky notes with affirmations on your bathroom mirror, fridge, or anywhere you'll see them throughout the day. These visual cues can serve as instant boosts of positivity.

Meditative Affirmations: Combine affirmations with your meditation or relaxation practices. Focusing on positive statements during these moments of quiet can deepen their impact.

Affirmation Journal: Keep a journal dedicated to your affirmations and reflections on how they make you feel. Writing affirmations down can reinforce their power and help you track your emotional journey through pregnancy.

Positive affirmations are more than just words; they're a practice of nurturing and empowering yourself from within. By regularly reminding yourself of your strength, capabilities, and the love surrounding you and your baby, you cultivate an environment where both you and your baby can thrive emotionally and physically. This practice of self-affirmation throughout pregnancy lays the foundation for a journey filled with confidence, joy, and profound connection.

The Impact

The incorporation of spiritual practices such as mindfulness, gratitude, and positive affirmations into the routine of an expectant mother plays a crucial role in creating a nurturing and healthy environment for both the mother and the baby. Let's explore the impact of these practices in more detail:

Reducing Stress

The journey of pregnancy, while beautiful, can also be fraught with anxieties and concerns about the future. Engaging in mindfulness exercises helps center thoughts in the present moment, significantly reducing stress levels. This reduction in stress is not just beneficial for the mother's mental health; it directly impacts the baby's development in a positive way. Lower stress levels are associated with fewer complications during pregnancy and can lead to a smoother, healthier gestation period.

Emotional Health

The power of gratitude in transforming one's outlook on life cannot be overstated. By focusing on the positives and cultivating a habit of thankfulness, expectant mothers can navigate the emotional rollercoaster of pregnancy with more resilience and joy. This positive emotional state is essential not just for the mother's well-being but also for creating a peaceful environment for the baby. Emotional health during pregnancy is closely linked to reduced risks of postpartum depression, making the practice of gratitude a valuable tool for expectant mothers.

Bonding with Your Baby

Positive affirmations are a powerful means of building a connection with the unborn child. Speaking words of love and strength to the baby, or simply thinking positively about the baby's health and the future, can foster a deep bond even before birth. This practice of affirmations helps in visualizing a healthy pregnancy and delivery, setting the stage for a strong emotional connection with the baby.

Physical Health

The benefits of these spiritual practices extend to physical health as well. Reduced stress and a positive mindset have been shown to contribute to better outcomes in pregnancy, including lower blood pressure, reduced risk of gestational diabetes, and healthier birth weights. Furthermore, the practice of mindfulness and gratitude can encourage healthier lifestyle choices, such as better nutrition and more consistent prenatal care, which directly benefit physical health.

Simple Ways to Incorporate These Practices

Incorporating these spiritual practices into daily life can be both simple and profound. Starting the day with a few moments of mindful breathing can set a positive tone for the rest of the day. Keeping a gratitude journal or simply reflecting on a few positive things each night before bed can cultivate a mindset of thankfulness. Repeating positive affirmations during times of stress or uncertainty can reinforce strength and positivity.

Incorporating Spiritual Practices into Daily Life

Incorporating spiritual practices into daily life during pregnancy can significantly enhance your journey, making it more peaceful, meaningful, and joyful. Here are some practical strategies for embedding mindfulness, gratitude, and positive affirmations into your routine:

Mindfulness in Daily Activities

Mindful Breathing: Start your day with a few minutes of mindful breathing. This can be done before getting out of bed, helping to center your thoughts and calm your mind for the day ahead.

Eating Mindfully: Turn meals into a practice of mindfulness by eating slowly and savoring each bite. Pay attention to the flavors, textures, and the nourishment your body is receiving.

Mindful Movement: Incorporate gentle movements, such as prenatal yoga or a short walk, into your routine. Focus on how your body feels with each movement and breath, enhancing your connection with your body and baby.

Cultivating Gratitude

Gratitude Journal: Keep a journal to jot down things you are grateful for each day. These could range from small pleasures to significant events, helping shift your focus to the positive aspects of your life.

Gratitude Moments: Throughout the day, pause to acknowledge and appreciate moments of beauty or kindness. This could be a supportive conversation, a comfortable moment of rest, or simply the feeling of your baby moving.

Sharing Gratitude: Share your grateful moments with your partner or a friend. This not only amplifies your positive feelings but also strengthens your relationships by focusing on positive interactions.

Practicing Positive Affirmations

Daily Affirmations: Create a list of affirmations that resonate with you, such as "I am capable of a healthy pregnancy" or "Every day, my baby and I are getting stronger." Repeat these affirmations to yourself each morning or whenever you need a confidence boost.

Affirmation Reminders: Place sticky notes with your affirmations in places you'll see them throughout the day, such as on the bathroom mirror or the refrigerator. These visual cues can serve as quick reminders of your strength and positivity.

Visualization: Combine your affirmations with visualization. Imagine yourself having a healthy pregnancy and delivery, and visualize a strong, positive future with your baby. This practice can deepen the impact of your affirmations, making them more meaningful and powerful.

Integration into Routine

Set Aside Time: Dedicate specific times in your routine for these practices. Early morning or before bed are often quiet moments ideal for reflection and mindfulness.

Be Flexible: Your energy levels and needs may change day by day. Be flexible with your practices, adapting them to how you feel and what you need most at any given time.

Involve Your Support Network: Share some of these practices with your partner or family members. Practising mindfulness or expressing gratitude together can enhance your connection and provide mutual support.

Incorporating these spiritual practices into your daily life during pregnancy isn't about adding more tasks to your day but about enriching the moments you already have. By embedding mindfulness, gratitude, and positive affirmations into your routine, you create a nurturing environment for yourself and your baby, fostering well-being, connection, and joy throughout your pregnancy journey.

Prayer

Prayer, or 'prarthana' as it's known from the Sanskrit words 'pro' and 'artha', translates to a heartfelt plea. It's an act where we reach out to God with a deep and passionate desire, seeking something with earnestness. This act of praying isn't just a request; it embodies our respect, faith, and devotion towards the divine. It's a humble acknowledgment of our limitations and an expression of our trust in a power greater than ourselves. In essence, prayer is a way to diminish our ego and expand our faith, guiding us towards a more spiritual and hopeful existence.

Understanding Prayer

Prayer serves as a fundamental connection between us and God, acting as a vital component of spiritual life. As noted by Hendry in 1972, prayer is not just a part of theology; it's a direct path to experiencing God's presence in our lives. William James, in 1902, beautifully captured the essence of prayer by describing it as "the very soul and essence of religion." This underscores the profound impact and importance of prayer in forging a deep, personal relationship with the Divine.

The Dual Nature of Prayer

The experience of connecting with God through prayer is similar to the two inseparable sides of a coin, highlighting the profound bond between the Divine and humanity. Van der Merwe in 2018 articulated that neither God nor humans are complete without this connection. Through prayer, we not only seek to bridge the gap between our earthly existence and the divine but also to understand our place within this vast universe. It's through this sacred conversation that we find solace, guidance, and a sense of belonging.

The Impact of Prayer During Pregnancy

Source of Positivity: For an expectant mother, moments of prayer can be a sanctuary of positivity. Amidst the whirlwind of emotions and physical changes, prayer offers a peaceful space to focus on the joy of creating new life. This positivity radiates within, helping to maintain an optimistic outlook which is beneficial for both mother and baby.

Spiritual Growth: Pregnancy is a transformative journey not just physically but spiritually as well. Regular prayer during this time can deepen a mother's spiritual awareness, helping her connect with the profound experience of bringing a new soul into the world. This spiritual connection can bring a sense of fulfillment and purpose, enriching the pregnancy journey.

Hope and Resilience: The path of pregnancy can sometimes be challenging. Prayer instills hope and cultivates resilience, providing the inner strength needed to navigate uncertainties or difficulties. It's a reminder that you are not alone, offering solace and support through faith.

Connection: Prayer during pregnancy strengthens the bond between mother, baby, and the Divine. It also nurtures connections with family, friends, and even oneself, fostering a supportive community around the pregnancy. This sense of belonging and understanding is invaluable, creating a nurturing environment for both emotional and spiritual growth.

Incorporating Prayer into Pregnancy

Integrating prayer into your pregnancy journey can be beautifully simple and deeply personal:

Quiet Moments: Dedicate a few quiet moments each day to prayer. This could be in the morning as you start your day, in the evening as you reflect, or any time you feel the need for peace and connection.

Gratitude Prayers: Use prayer as a way to express gratitude for the new life growing inside you. Acknowledging the miracle of pregnancy can enhance your sense of wonder and appreciation.

Guidance and Support: Seek guidance and support through prayer, asking for strength, health, and protection for you and your baby. This can be comforting and reassuring, especially during moments of worry.

Meditative Prayer: Combine prayer with meditation, focusing on your connection with your baby. This can be a time to share love, hopes, and dreams with your unborn child, strengthening the bond before birth.

Benefits of Prayer

The good things that come from praying, especially when you're expecting a baby, cover a lot of ground. Studies, like the one by Levine in 2001, show that praying can make you healthier, give you a better quality of life, and make you feel less stressed. This means praying can be a big help when you're dealing with all the changes and feelings that come with pregnancy.

Prayer is a way we talk and connect, covering everything from traditional religious prayers to just talking to what you believe in quietly and meditating. Baesler and Ladd (2009), and Plante (2010) talk about how important this communication is. For someone who's pregnant, praying can be a source of power. It helps with getting through tough parts of pregnancy and making big health decisions. It's more than just a way to handle hard stuff; it gives you a sense of meaning, hope, and control over your life.

Praying while you're pregnant can bring you a deep peace and help you accept the big changes coming your way. This peace is key to getting through pregnancy in a good way. Praying helps cut down on stress and worry, which is great for both the mom and the baby. Feeling hopeful and looking at life positively can make you emotionally stronger and ready to face whatever comes.

Prayer also helps you keep your cool when things get tough. It teaches you to be patient, to think about others, and to understand yourself better by thinking deeply about your life. These are all important as you get ready to become a mom.

Praying also makes your relationships stronger. It makes you more understanding and caring towards other people. This is really helpful during pregnancy when you need your friends and family around you. Plus, praying makes you more aware of the world around you and helps you live by your values, making your journey to becoming a parent more meaningful.

In short, praying while you're pregnant does a lot more than just connect you spiritually. It looks after your mind, body, and heart, creating a calm, clear, and loving space as you get ready for the new life you're bringing into the world. It shows just how much your spiritual health can boost your physical health, making your time being pregnant richer and more filled with joy.

Action Item

Set aside 10 minutes each day for a spiritual practice that resonates with you, such as prayer, meditation, or reading inspirational texts.

Chapter 5

"Nurturing Wellness: The Power of Exercise and Yoga During Pregnancy"

Movement and Breath

What are movement and breath? At their core, movement and breath are fundamental elements of life, especially during pregnancy. Movement refers to physical activity, the act of keeping your body active and engaged through various exercises or practices. It's about using your muscles, stretching, and staying flexible, which is essential for a healthy pregnancy. Breath, on the other hand, involves focusing on how you breathe, using techniques to control and make the most of each breath. It's about drawing in air in a way that nourishes both your body and your baby, supporting your health and well-being.

Together, movement and breath play a vital role during pregnancy. They're not just about staying fit or relaxed; they're about creating a strong, healthy environment for your baby to grow. Engaging in regular physical activity and practicing mindful breathing can enhance your pregnancy experience, making it healthier and more joyful. These practices support your body's changes, prepare you for childbirth, and help you find balance and calm as you navigate the journey of pregnancy.

Movement in Pregnancy

Movement, or physical activity, during pregnancy isn't just about exercise in the conventional sense. It encompasses any form of bodily motion that keeps you active—be it walking, swimming, prenatal yoga, or simply stretching. The essence of movement lies in its ability to engage and strengthen the body's muscles, enhancing flexibility and endurance. These qualities are crucial as your body adapts to carry the growing weight of your baby.

Regular movement helps in various ways:

Enhances Circulation: Improved blood flow ensures that essential nutrients and oxygen are efficiently delivered to both the mother and the baby.

Prepares for Labor: Exercises targeting the pelvic floor muscles can play a significant role in preparing your body for the demands of labor and childbirth.

Alleviates Common Discomforts: By strengthening the back and improving posture, movement can reduce the prevalence of back pain, a common complaint during pregnancy.

Regulates Mood: The release of endorphins through exercise acts as a natural mood booster, helping to manage stress and anxiety.

Breath in Pregnancy

Breath, or the focus on breathing techniques, is equally vital. Proper breathing practices can significantly impact your and your baby's health by optimizing oxygen flow. Mindful breathing, such as deep abdominal breathing, encourages relaxation and stress reduction. It can also play a critical role during labor, helping to manage pain and maintain calm.

Benefits of focused breathing include:

Stress Reduction: Deep, controlled breathing activates the body's relaxation response, counteracting the stress hormones.

Oxygenates the Blood: Efficient breathing increases oxygen levels in the blood, crucial for the baby's development.

Enhances Emotional Connection: Mindful breathing can create moments of deep connection between the mother and the baby, fostering a sense of peace and bonding.

Integrating Movement and Breath

Integrating movement and breath into your pregnancy involves more than sporadic exercises. It's about creating a consistent routine that caters to your body's evolving needs. This might mean starting with gentle walks and prenatal yoga in the earlier months and focusing more on breathwork and pelvic floor exercises as you approach labor.

Listening to your body is key. Some days, a full workout might feel right; on others, a few stretches and deep breathing exercises might be all you need. The goal is to maintain a balance that keeps you physically active and mentally serene, ensuring a healthier, more vibrant pregnancy.

The Vital Role of Movement

The vital role of movement during pregnancy cannot be overstated. Engaging in physical activity is essential for maintaining a healthy pregnancy for several reasons.

Firstly, regular movement helps to enhance cardiovascular health, ensuring that both you and your baby receive ample oxygen and nutrients. This boost in circulation also aids in preventing common pregnancy discomforts, such as swelling and varicose veins, by promoting blood flow throughout the body.

Additionally, staying active strengthens the muscles needed for labor and delivery. Exercises that focus on the pelvic floor, for instance, can prepare your body for the birthing process, potentially leading to a smoother labor and recovery. Strengthening your core, back, and legs also helps in accommodating the growing weight of your baby, which can alleviate back pain and improve posture.

Physical activity during pregnancy has been shown to regulate emotional well-being too. It releases endorphins, which are natural mood elevators, helping to reduce feelings of stress and anxiety. This emotional regulation is vital, as the well-being of the mother directly impacts the health of the developing baby.

Moreover, engaging in regular exercise can help manage gestational weight gain within healthy limits, reducing the risk of gestational diabetes and preeclampsia. It's not about maintaining fitness levels or body image but about nurturing a healthy environment for your baby to grow.

It's important, however, to choose safe, pregnancy-appropriate activities and to consult with a healthcare provider before starting any new exercise routine. The goal is to stay active and healthy, listening to your body's needs and adapting as your pregnancy progresses. This commitment to movement is a beautiful way to honor your body's incredible journey and to support your baby's development with every step.

The Power of Breath

The power of breath during pregnancy is profound and multifaceted, significantly impacting both maternal and baby's health. Focused breathing, or the practice of consciously controlling your breath, is more than a relaxation technique; it's a vital tool for nurturing life.

For the Mother

Stress Reduction: Pregnancy can be a time of heightened emotions and stress. Focused breathing activates the parasympathetic nervous system, which slows the heart rate and lowers blood pressure, creating a sense of calm and reducing stress. This not only improves the mother's emotional well-being but also contributes to a healthier pregnancy.

Pain Management: During labor, focused breathing techniques can be invaluable for managing discomfort. By concentrating on your breath, you can divert attention from pain, using rhythm and depth of breathing as a natural pain relief tool. This can make the birthing process more manageable and less intimidating.

Improved Oxygenation: Deep breathing increases oxygen levels in the bloodstream. This is beneficial for the mother's body, aiding in energy production and overall vitality. An oxygen-rich environment also supports the baby's development and growth.

Emotional Bonding: Taking time for focused breathing allows for moments of quiet connection with the baby. These peaceful interludes can enhance the emotional bond between mother and baby, fostering a sense of closeness and anticipation for the life they will share.

For the Baby

Optimal Development: The increased oxygenation resulting from the mother's focused breathing benefits the baby directly. Oxygen is crucial for fetal development, supporting everything from brain growth to the maturation of vital organs.

Stress Reduction: The baby is sensitive to the mother's emotional state. A calm and relaxed mother, achieved through focused breathing, can contribute to a serene environment for the baby, potentially reducing stress impacts on the baby's development.

Healthy Birth Outcome: Practices that incorporate focused breathing, such as prenatal yoga or meditation, have been associated with healthier birth outcomes. This includes reduced chances of preterm labor and improved birth weights, partly due to the overall stress-reducing, health-enhancing benefits of these practices.

Incorporating Focused Breathing

Integrating focused breathing into daily life can be simple and adaptable to any schedule. It can involve dedicating a few minutes each morning to deep breathing exercises, using breathing techniques as a relaxation tool before bed, or practicing breath control as part of a prenatal yoga routine. The key is consistency and making these practices a regular part of your pregnancy care.

In essence, the power of breath during pregnancy is a testament to the simple yet profound impact that breathing can have on both mother and baby. By accepting focused breathing practices, expectant mothers can enhance their well-being, prepare for childbirth, and provide a nurturing environment for their developing baby, underscoring the beautiful interconnectedness of mother and child through the act of breathing.

Finding Your Movement

Finding the right kind of movement during pregnancy is key to maintaining health and well-being for both you and your baby. It's about discovering physical activities that are safe, enjoyable, and beneficial throughout the various stages of pregnancy. Here's a look at some recommended exercises tailored for expectant mothers:

Walking

Walking is a simple yet effective exercise for expectant mothers. It's low impact, can be done almost anywhere, and is easily adjusted to your fitness level. Regular walks can help maintain cardiovascular health, manage weight gain, and improve mood.

Swimming and Water Aerobics

Water provides natural resistance and supports your body, making swimming and water aerobics excellent choices for pregnancy. These activities minimize the strain on your joints and back while providing a good cardiovascular workout.

Prenatal Yoga

Prenatal yoga focuses on gentle stretching, controlled breathing, and relaxation techniques. It's designed to address the specific needs of pregnant women, such as relieving lower back pain and enhancing flexibility, which can be beneficial during childbirth.

Stationary Cycling

Stationary cycling is another safe option for pregnancy. It allows for cardiovascular exercise without the risk of falling. Adjusting the intensity is straightforward, making it suitable for all stages of pregnancy.

Low-Impact Aerobics

Low-impact aerobics classes designed for pregnant women can provide a fun way to stay active. These classes focus on maintaining heart health without putting too much stress on your joints.

Strength Training

Moderate strength training, using light weights or bodyweight exercises, can help maintain muscle tone during pregnancy. It's important to focus on proper form and possibly modify exercises as your pregnancy progresses.

Guidelines for Safe Exercise During Pregnancy

Consult with a Healthcare Provider: Before starting any new exercise regimen, it's essential to talk with your healthcare provider, especially if you have any pregnancy-related conditions or concerns.

Stay Hydrated: Drink plenty of water before, during, and after exercising to stay hydrated.

Avoid Overexertion: Listen to your body and avoid pushing yourself too hard. The goal is to stay active and healthy, not to reach peak fitness levels.

Monitor Your Heart Rate: Keep your heart rate at a safe level for pregnancy. Your healthcare provider can offer specific guidelines based on your individual health.

Pay Attention to Your Body: If you feel dizzy, short of breath, or experience any pain, stop exercising and consult your healthcare provider.

Finding your movement during pregnancy is about more than just staying fit; it's a way to enhance your overall health and prepare your body for the journey ahead. By choosing safe, pregnancy-appropriate exercises, you can enjoy an active pregnancy and support your body's well-being as you prepare for the arrival of your baby.

Yoga and Pranayama

"Yama, Niyama, Asana, Pranayama, Pratyahara, Dharana, Dhyana and Samadhi are the eight limbs.
– "Patanjala Yoga Darshan"

Yoga

Yoga is a practice rooted in ancient wisdom, originating from the Sanskrit word "Yuj," which means "to join." It's described in the Bhagavad Gita as "yogh karmasu kaushlam," highlighting its essence as the art of skillfully living life. Yoga brings harmony to the body, mind, and soul, making it a comprehensive approach to well-being.

The Importance of Yoga During Pregnancy

During pregnancy, yoga serves as a vital tool for maintaining health and fostering a sense of calm. It aids in ensuring a normal delivery by enhancing neuromuscular coordination and reducing the chances of prematurity by lowering stress-related cortisol levels. Additionally, the release of endorphin hormones during yoga practice helps balance the physical, mental, and emotional states of both mother and child.

Pregnancy brings with it a range of challenges, including back pain, constipation, anxiety, sleep disturbances, leg swelling, gestational diabetes, acidity, morning sickness, decreased appetite, fatigue, body aches, and pregnancy-induced hypertension. Yoga offers a gentle yet effective way to address and alleviate these issues.

By incorporating yoga into their routine, expectant mothers can significantly reduce the risks of preterm labor, intrauterine growth retardation (IUGR), preeclampsia, gestational diabetes (GDM), pelvic pain, stress, anxiety, and depression.

Precautions During Exercise and Yoga

Safety is paramount when practicing yoga during pregnancy. It's crucial to:

- Consult a doctor before beginning any new exercise regimen.

- Exercise caution if you have high blood pressure, low placental implantation, bleeding during pregnancy, cervical incompetence, or are expecting twins.

- Avoid asanas that exert pressure on the abdomen and those that involve hard postures or pressure on the lower abdomen.

- During the first trimester, focus on walking and meditation instead of yoga.

Preparation Before Starting Yoga and Exercise

For the best experience, consider the following guidelines:

- Practice yoga in the early morning on an empty stomach for optimal benefits.

- Begin your session after attending to natural calls.

- If possible, choose a clean, open-air environment for your practice.

- Wear clean, loose-fitting clothing.

- Wait 30-45 minutes after consuming liquids and 3-4 hours after meals before practicing yoga.

- Use a thick carpet for comfort and safety.

- Avoid overstretching. Stay within your comfort zone and be mindful of your breath, living in the present moment.

Advantages of Yoga During Pregnancy

Yoga during pregnancy offers numerous benefits:

- Increases flexibility in pelvic muscles.

- Strengthens bones.

- Relieves tension around the cervix.

- Balances the endocrine system.

- Retones and stretches waist and pelvic muscles that weaken during and after pregnancy.

Exercise Benefits

Incorporating stretching into your daily routine can enhance fitness, reduce pregnancy-related discomforts, and prepare your body for labor. These gentle exercises are designed to relieve aches and improve your overall pregnancy experience.

By adopting yoga and incorporating recommended exercises into your pregnancy journey, you engage in a holistic practice that not only prepares your body for childbirth but also supports your overall well-being, creating a positive and nurturing environment for your growing baby.

Back Stretching Exercises During Pregnancy

1. *Cat-Cow Pose (Marjaryasana to Bitilasana)*

The Cat-Cow Pose, known as Marjaryasana to Bitilasana in yoga, is a wonderfully supportive exercise for expectant mothers. This pose focuses on gently strengthening the muscles while maintaining flexibility in the lower back and abdomen, areas that are crucial during pregnancy. It's a soothing exercise that not only relieves tension but also enhances spinal mobility and promotes healthy blood circulation. Here's a simple guide on how to incorporate the Cat-Cow stretch into your routine:

Instructions for Cat-Cow Pose:

Starting Position: Begin by positioning yourself on all fours on a stable, comfortable surface. Ensure your hands are directly under your shoulders, spread at shoulder width, and your knees are set apart at hip width. This stable base is important for your balance and to ensure the exercise is effective and safe.

Cow Pose (Bitilasana):

- Inhale deeply, and as you do, slowly lower your belly towards the mat, creating a gentle arch in your lower back.

- Lift your head and tailbone upwards, letting your gaze drift upwards. This position encourages a nice stretch across your abdomen and engages your back muscles lightly.

Cat Pose (Marjaryasana):

- As you exhale, begin to draw your chin towards your chest, rounding your spine upwards like a cat stretching.

- Gently tuck your tailbone under as you push the middle of your back towards the ceiling, creating an arch.

- This motion helps to release tension in your back and neck, providing relief and improving flexibility.

Flowing Between Poses:

- Continue to flow smoothly between the Cow Pose and the Cat Pose, matching your movement with your breath. Inhale as you move into Cow Pose and exhale into Cat Pose.

- Aim to continue this fluid movement for up to one minute, focusing on the rhythm of your breath and the movement of your spine.

Additional Tips:

- For added comfort, especially as your pregnancy progresses, place a folded blanket under your knees. This extra cushioning helps protect your joints and makes it easier to maintain the pose for longer periods.

- Always listen to your body. If you experience any discomfort, adjust your stance or reduce the range of motion. The goal is gentle stretching and relaxation, not strain.

2. Child's Pose (Balasana)

The Child's Pose, or Balasana, is a deeply restorative yoga pose that offers a gentle stretch for the back, hips, and thighs—areas that often carry tension during pregnancy. This pose is particularly beneficial for easing back pain, as it stretches the lower back, chest, and shoulders, while also promoting flexibility in the spine, hips, and thighs. Here's how to safely enjoy the benefits of the Child's Pose during pregnancy:

Instructions for Child's Pose:

- **Starting Position:** Position yourself on all fours on a comfortable, supportive surface. This initial stance ensures stability as you move into the pose.

- **Setting Your Base:** Gently spread your knees apart while keeping your big toes touching. This adjustment provides room for your belly and enhances the stretch in your hips and thighs.

Lowering Into the Pose:

- Gradually lower your hips back towards your heels. This motion should be smooth and controlled, focusing on the stretch it provides.

- Extend your arms forward on the floor, allowing your upper body to relax and stretch out. This extension not only aids in deepening the stretch but also helps in releasing tension in your shoulders and neck.

Breathing:

- Take a deep breath in, filling your lungs and back with air. The act of deep breathing enhances relaxation and increases the stretch's benefits.

- Hold the pose for up to one minute, focusing on deep, steady breaths. This duration allows your body to relax into the pose and maximizes its benefits.

Additional Comfort Measures:

- For extra support, especially if you have sensitive knees or need additional comfort for your forehead, place a cushion or folded blanket where needed. A cushion under your forehead can help if reaching the floor is uncomfortable, while a blanket under the knees can protect against pressure and discomfort.

- If your belly needs more space or if you experience knee discomfort, try widening your toes further apart. This simple adjustment can make a significant difference in how the pose feels, allowing for a more personalized stretch that accommodates your body's needs during pregnancy.

3. *Modified Half Pigeon Pose*

The modified pigeon pose is a fantastic exercise for expectant mothers experiencing lower back pain. This variation, suited for pregnancy, focuses on relaxing the piriformis muscle located in the glutes. Stretching this small but significant muscle can significantly alleviate tightness and discomfort in the lower back area. Here's how to perform this gentle stretch safely:

Instructions for Modified Pigeon Pose:

- **Starting Position:** Begin by sitting comfortably on a chair, ensuring it's stable and at a height where your feet can rest flat on the ground. This stable base is essential for maintaining balance and ensuring the effectiveness of the stretch.

Creating the "4" Shape:

- Carefully lift one foot and place it over the knee of your opposite leg. Arrange your legs to form the shape of the number "4". This position starts the process of targeting the piriformis muscle.

Initiating the Stretch:

- Take a deep breath in. As you exhale slowly, gently lean your upper body forward from your hips. It's important to keep your back straight to avoid any strain and maximize the stretch in the intended areas.

- Continue leaning forward until you feel a stretch in your lower back and the buttock of the crossed leg. This sensation indicates that the piriformis muscle is being effectively stretched.

Holding the Pose:

- Once you find a comfortable stretch, hold the position for about 30 seconds. This duration allows the muscles to relax and stretch adequately.

- Remember to breathe normally throughout the hold, as this will help deepen the stretch and promote relaxation.

Repeating on the Other Side:

- Gently return to your starting position and switch legs to repeat the stretch on the other side. This ensures that both sides of your body receive equal attention and benefit from the exercise.

Additional Tips:

- This exercise is particularly beneficial for those who suffer from lower back pain during pregnancy. The chair provides support and makes it easier to maintain balance, making this stretch safe and accessible.

- Always listen to your body. If you experience any discomfort beyond a gentle stretch, adjust your position or discontinue the exercise.

- Consistency is key. Regularly incorporating this modified pigeon pose into your routine can contribute significantly to reducing lower back pain and improving your pregnancy experience.

Hip Stretching Exercises During Pregnancy

1. Easy Pose (Sukhasana)

This particular stretching exercise is designed to nurture expectant mothers by elongating the spine, creating space in the hips, and enhancing mental focus. Here's how you can incorporate this beneficial stretch into your daily routine:

Instructions for the Stretch:

Setting the Foundation:

- Begin by sitting on the edge of a cushion or folded blanket. This slight elevation allows your pelvis to tilt forward naturally, encouraging a healthy posture.

Finding Your Seat:

- Cross your legs in a way that feels natural and comfortable for you, with either the right or left leg in front. This seated position helps to open your hips gently, accommodating your growing baby while maintaining comfort.

Hand Position and Focus:

- Place your hands in a position that feels restful, whether on your knees or in your lap. Close your eyes to turn your attention inward, preparing for deep breathing.

Breathing:

- Inhale deeply, filling your lungs and expanding your ribcage. Hold this breath for up to one minute, although even a few seconds can be beneficial if that's what feels comfortable to you.

- As you exhale, imagine releasing any tension or stress from your body and mind.

Repetition:

- After exhaling, take a moment and then repeat the deep breathing cycle, focusing on the calm and space each breath brings to your body.

Enhancing Comfort:

- For added support to your spine, consider practicing with your back against a wall. This can help maintain a straight, elongated spine without straining.

- If you plan to stay in this pose for an extended period, such as during meditation, placing cushions or blankets under your knees can provide additional support and comfort, ensuring that you can maintain the pose without discomfort.

2. Bridge Pose (Setu Bandha Sarvangasana)

The bridge pose is a gentle yet effective exercise for expectant mothers, focusing on stretching the hip flexors while simultaneously strengthening the lower back, abs, and glutes. It's particularly beneficial for alleviating discomfort in the hips and lower back, common areas of tension during pregnancy. Here's how to safely perform the bridge pose:

Instructions for the Bridge Pose:

Starting Position:

- Begin by lying on your back on a comfortable surface, ensuring your knees are bent and your feet are flat on the floor. Your feet should be set hip-width apart to provide stable support.

Arm Positioning:

- Extend your arms straight alongside your body. If your flexibility allows, adjust your leg position so your fingers can lightly touch the backs of your heels. This alignment helps ensure proper form as you move into the pose.

Lifting Into the Pose:

- As you inhale, gently lift your hips towards the ceiling. Engage your glutes to support the lift, keeping a mindful eye on your knees to ensure they don't bow outward.

Holding the Pose:

- Hold this lifted position for a few breaths, focusing on the stretch and strength being built in your hips, back, and abdominal muscles.

Returning to Start:

- On an exhale, carefully roll your spine back down to the ground, returning to your starting position.

Repetition:

- Repeat this lifting and lowering motion ten times, moving smoothly and coordinating each movement with your breath.

Enhancing the Pose:

- For an added challenge and to ensure proper alignment, place a yoga block between your inner thighs. By squeezing the block gently, you activate the thigh stabilisers, which not only enhance the effectiveness of the exercise but also ensure your legs maintain proper alignment throughout the pose.

3. Butterfly Pose (Baddha Konasana)

The butterfly pose, known for its gentle opening and stretching of the hips, is an excellent exercise for expectant mothers aiming to enhance flexibility and prepare their bodies for labor. This pose not only promotes blood circulation and stimulates the digestive system but also relaxes the muscles, specifically targeting the lower back, hips, and inner thighs. Here's how to incorporate the butterfly pose into your prenatal routine:

Instructions for Butterfly Pose:

Finding Your Base:

- Start by sitting on the edge of a cushion or folded blanket. This slight elevation helps tilt your pelvis forward, aligning your spine more naturally for the stretch.

Positioning Your Feet:

- Bring the soles of your feet together in front of you, allowing your knees to fall gently to the sides. The closer you draw your feet toward your hips, the deeper the stretch will be in your inner thighs and hips.

Spinal Alignment:

- Focus on lengthening your spine upwards, creating a sense of lift and openness through your torso. This posture ensures you're stretching effectively while protecting your back.

Hand Placement:

- Gently rest your hands on your ankles or shins. This position helps maintain balance and supports the stretch without straining.

Holding the Pose:

- Maintain this pose for up to a minute, concentrating on deep, steady breaths to help relax into the stretch.

- Gently release and repeat the pose 2-4 times, allowing each repetition to deepen the stretch and increase flexibility.

Enhancing Comfort and Support:

- For additional support, especially if you find sitting on the floor challenging, position your back against a wall. This can help you maintain an upright spine without extra effort.

- Placing cushions or folded blankets under your knees or thighs can provide support and reduce strain, particularly helpful if you experience discomfort in the stretch.

4. Garland pose (Malasana)

The deep squat, often recognized for its ability to extensively open the hips, is another valuable exercise for expectant mothers. This posture not only aids in improving digestion but is also instrumental in preparing the body for labor and delivery by enhancing flexibility and strength in the pelvic area. Here's how to safely execute the deep squat:

Instructions for Deep Squat:

Starting Position:

- Begin standing with your feet set slightly wider than hip-width apart, toes pointing outward. This stance is crucial for balance and allows for a deeper squat while accommodating your growing belly.

Entering the Squat:

- Gradually bend your knees, lowering your hips towards the floor as if sitting back into a chair. Keep the movement slow and controlled to prevent strain.

Heel Position:

- Depending on your balance and comfort, you can either keep your heels lifted off the floor or flat against it. If lifting, try to maintain as much stability as possible.

Upper Body Alignment:

- Once in the squat, bring your palms together at the center of your chest in a prayer position. Use your elbows to gently press against the inside of your knees, aiding in opening your hips further.

Holding the Pose:

- Aim to maintain this position for up to 30 seconds, breathing deeply to help relax into the stretch. The duration can be adjusted based on your comfort level.

Repetition:

- Carefully release from the squat and stand. Repeat the exercise, aiming for consistency in form and depth with each repetition.

Modifications for Support and Safety:

- For added support, especially useful if maintaining balance becomes challenging, consider performing the squat against a wall. This provides a sturdy backrest that can help you sustain the pose with less effort.

- Alternatively, sitting on a block or a stack of cushions can offer a similar benefit by reducing the distance you need to squat, making the pose more accessible while still reaping the hip-opening benefits.

- It's important to note that if you have a history of prolapse or have been advised against deep squats by your healthcare provider, it's best to avoid this exercise. Always prioritize safety and listen to your body's signals.

5. Lunge Pose

This pose, designed to ease tightness in the hip flexors, is especially beneficial during pregnancy. As the body adapts to changes in pelvic position, the muscles along the front of your hip can often tighten, leading to discomfort. Here's a gentle way to stretch these muscles and find some relief:

Instructions for the Hip Flexor Stretch:

Preparing Your Space:

- Start by kneeling on a comfortable surface. To protect your knees, consider placing a pillow or folded blanket beneath them for extra cushioning.

Entering the Stretch:

- Carefully step one foot forward, planting it flat on the ground so that both your knee and hip form 90-degree angles. This positioning is crucial for targeting the hip flexors effectively.

Deepening the Stretch:

- As you exhale, gently lean into your front leg, distributing your weight forward. This motion will begin to stretch the hip flexor of your back leg.

- To intensify the stretch, subtly rotate your back hip forward. Continue until you feel a stretch through the front of your hip and thigh.

Holding the Pose:

- Hold this position for 30 seconds, breathing deeply and evenly as you do. The duration allows the muscle to slowly relax and stretch, maximizing the benefit.

Switching Sides:

- Carefully come out of the pose, switch legs, and repeat the stretch on the opposite side to ensure both hips are equally worked.

Additional Support:

- If balancing becomes a challenge, feel free to stabilize yourself by placing a hand on a nearby wall or chair. This support can help you maintain the pose without straining.

- The use of a pillow under your knees is a thoughtful way to make this exercise more comfortable, especially as your pregnancy progresses and your body requires extra care.

Legs Stretching Exercises During Pregnancy

1. Standing Forward Bend (Uttanasana)

The Standing Forward Bend, or Uttanasana, is a rejuvenating yoga pose that offers several benefits, making it particularly useful during pregnancy. It focuses on strengthening the thighs and knees while maintaining spinal flexibility. Additionally, this pose is known for its ability to relieve tension and foster a sense of inner calm. Here's how to safely perform the Standing Forward Bend during pregnancy:

Instructions for Standing Forward Bend:

Starting Position:

- Begin by standing with your feet slightly wider than hip-distance apart. This wider stance provides a stable base and accommodates your growing belly comfortably.

Folding Forward:

- Gently hinge your hips to fold forward, leading with your chest to keep the spine long. Keeping a slight bend in your knees helps to relieve pressure on the lower back and makes the pose more accessible during pregnancy.

Hand Placement:

- Depending on your flexibility, place your hands on the floor, a yoga block, or simply let them dangle toward the ground. Using a block can help bring the ground closer to you, making the pose more comfortable.

Holding the Pose:

- Aim to hold the pose for up to 30 seconds, breathing deeply throughout. The duration allows your body to gradually release into the stretch, enhancing its benefits.

Support Option:

- For additional support, especially useful if you're seeking extra balance or have concerns about falling, practice this pose in front of a wall. The wall can serve as a reassuring support for your hands or shoulders.

Modifications and Tips:

- Practicing the Standing Forward Bend in front of a wall provides not only physical support but also a sense of safety as you deepen into the pose.

- Always listen to your body's cues. If you feel any discomfort, especially in the back or hamstrings, ease up on the intensity of the bend.

- Maintaining a slight bend in the knees not only protects the lower back but also ensures the stretch remains gentle on the hamstrings, making the pose more beneficial during pregnancy.

2. Downward Dog Pose (Adho mukha svana-sana)

The Downward Dog Pose, or Adho Mukha Svanasana, is a foundational yoga posture that offers a comprehensive stretch across the entire back, from the neck down to the heels. Regarded as a gentle inversion, this pose uniquely positions the body to allow oxygen-rich blood to flow toward the brain, enhancing overall circulation and providing a refreshing energy boost. Here's how to integrate the Downward Dog Pose into your prenatal yoga practice safely:

Instructions for Downward Dog Pose:

Starting Position:

- Begin on all fours, ensuring your hands are set shoulder-width apart and your knees are hip-width apart for a stable foundation. Position your hands slightly in front of your shoulders and align your knees directly under your hips.

Entering the Pose:

- Curl your toes under and press firmly through your palms, spreading your fingers for added stability. Gently lift your hips up and back, transitioning your body into an inverted "V" shape.

Refining the Pose:

- Actively push the floor away with your hands, focusing on lifting your pelvis towards the ceiling. Engage your upper arm triceps to stabilize your form, ensuring a balanced distribution of weight.

Maintaining the Pose:

- Aim to hold this position for about a minute, allowing your breath to flow naturally. This duration lets your body fully benefit from the stretch and inversion.

Transitioning Out:

- As you exhale, softly bend your knees and transition back into Child's Pose. This counterpose allows for a moment of rest and recentering.

Modifications and Considerations:

- For those experiencing nausea, heartburn, or wrist pain, it's advisable to skip the Downward Dog Pose. Always listen to your body and consult with your healthcare provider or a prenatal yoga instructor for alternatives that suit your specific needs.

- Using yoga blocks under your hands can alleviate pressure on the wrists and help maintain proper alignment.

- Remember, the goal of prenatal yoga is to enhance your comfort and well-being. Adjusting the pose to meet your body's changing needs throughout pregnancy is not only recommended but encouraged.

Adding stretching exercises to your daily routine while pregnant is a great way to take care of yourself. It's important to listen to your body and take breaks whenever you feel like you need them.

Take Away

Before you start doing any new exercises, including stretching, you should talk to your doctor. This is really important if your pregnancy is considered high-risk, if you have any health issues, or if you haven't done much exercise before. Your doctor can help make sure that your exercise plan is safe for you and your baby.

Remember, stretching during pregnancy isn't just about staying in shape. It's also about feeling good and staying connected with your body as it changes. Always listen to your body, take it easy when you need to, and get advice from your doctor to keep you and your baby healthy.

Pranayama

"Pranayama" during pregnancy is about accepting the essence of breath and life energy, focusing on the gentle regulation of the breath rather than physical postures or asanas. Here's a simplified look into what makes pranayama an integral part of prenatal care:

Understanding Pranayama:

- Prana means "life force," and Ayam refers to "regulation" or "dimension." So, pranayama translates to the "regulation of life force."

- It's considered even more crucial than asana (physical yoga poses) during pregnancy because of its direct impact on both the mother's and baby's well-being.

The Practice:

- The key is to breathe slowly, deeply, and consciously, focusing on both inhalation and exhalation.

- Note: It's important not to hold your breath (avoid Kumbhak) during pregnancy, to ensure safety for both mother and child.

Scientific Benefits of Pranayama:

- **Increases Vitality and Immunity:** By enhancing oxygen supply and boosting positivity, pranayama prepares the body to fight off illnesses and maintain energy.

- **Improves Circulation:** Better blood flow eases common pregnancy complaints like constipation, acidity, and diabetes, and calms the nervous system.

- **Mental Health Benefits:** Regular practice can alleviate depression, stress, anxiety, and headaches, including migraines, contributing to a peaceful mind.

- **Purifies and Activates Energy Channels:** Pranayama cleanses the nadis (energy channels), ensuring the smooth flow of prana, essential for the well-being of both mother and fetus.

- **Happiness Hormone:** The practice encourages the release of serotonin, promoting happiness and contentment in both the mother and the developing baby.

Some pranayama practices that may be beneficial during pregnancy include:

1. Deep abdominal breathing

Deep abdominal breathing is a simple yet profoundly effective pranayama practice that can be particularly beneficial during pregnancy. This technique focuses on full, deep inhalations and exhalations, encouraging a sense of calm and relaxation while enhancing oxygen flow to both the mother and the baby. Here's how to incorporate deep abdominal breathing into your prenatal care routine:

How to Practise Deep Abdominal Breathing:

Find a Comfortable Position:

- Sit in a comfortable chair with good back support or on the floor with a cushion for support. Ensure your spine is straight but not tense.

Place Your Hands:

- Gently place one hand on your belly and the other on your chest. This will help you become more aware of the movement of your breath.

Inhale Deeply:

- Slowly inhale through your nose, allowing your belly to expand fully. Feel the hand on your belly rise as your breath fills the lower part of your lungs.

Exhale Slowly:

- Exhale gently through your mouth or nose, whichever feels more comfortable. As you exhale, feel your belly fall, and use the hand on your belly to help gently press out the remaining air.

Continue the Cycle:

- Repeat this breathing pattern for several minutes. Focus on making your inhalations and exhalations as smooth and steady as possible.

Benefits for Pregnant Mothers:

- **Stress Reduction:** Deep abdominal breathing helps to reduce stress levels by activating the body's natural relaxation response.

- **Improved Oxygenation:** By encouraging full breaths, this practice enhances oxygen supply to both the mother and the developing fetus, supporting healthy growth.

- **Lower Blood Pressure:** Regular practice can contribute to lower blood pressure by promoting relaxation and reducing stress hormones.

- **Digestive Health:** The gentle expansion and contraction of the abdomen can help stimulate digestion and alleviate discomfort.

- **Preparation for Labor:** Learning to control and focus on your breath can be an invaluable tool during labor, aiding in pain management and relaxation.

2. Nadi shodhan pranayama

Nadi Shodhan Pranayama, or alternate nostril breathing, enriched with the vibrations of the Gayatri Mahamantra, is a deeply nourishing practice during pregnancy. This technique aims to balance and cleanse the energy channels, or nadis, within the body, harmonizing the body's physical, mental, and spiritual dimensions. Here's a step-by-step guide to practicing Nadi Shodhan Pranayama during pregnancy:

Steps for Nadi Shodhan Pranayama with Gayatri Mahamantra:

Starting Position:

- Sit comfortably with your spine straight and shoulders relaxed. You can sit on a chair or on the floor with a cushion for support.

First Phase:

- Gently close your right nostril with your thumb and inhale deeply through your left nostril three times, focusing on visualizing the moon's calming energy in your navel area.

Second Phase:

- Using your fingers, close off your left nostril and exhale through your right nostril three times, concentrating on the sun's radiant energy in your navel area.

Balanced Breathing:

- Inhale evenly through both nostrils, then exhale gently through your mouth, envisioning any physical or mental disorders being expelled from your body.

Incorporating Gayatri Mahamantra:

- While practicing the breathing cycles, silently recite or mentally focus on the Gayatri Mahamantra, infusing your practice with its powerful spiritual energy.

Benefits of the Practice:

- Nadi Shodhan Pranayama balances the nervous system, offering relief in arthritis by stimulating the gastric fire and increasing appetite. It harmonizes the Ida and Pingala nadis, crucial for the holistic well-being of both mother and child.

- This pranayama aids in the physical, mental, and spiritual development of the baby in the womb and maintains a balanced body temperature.

Considerations During Pregnancy:

- Ensure you're in a comfortable seated position that does not strain your back or abdomen.

- Focus on gentle inhalations and exhalations without straining, especially when practicing pranayama with mantra meditation.

- Listen to your body's cues, and if any discomfort arises, gently pause your practice.

3. Bhramari pranayama

Bhramari Pranayama, also known as the Humming Bee Breath, is a soothing and effective breathing technique ideal for pregnant women. It's named after the black Indian bee called Bhramari because of the humming sound produced during the practice, resembling the gentle buzz of a bee. This pranayama brings a multitude of benefits, making it a valuable addition to your prenatal routine.

Benefits of Bhramari Pranayama:

- **Reduces Risk of Preeclampsia:** Regular practice can help decrease the chances of developing preeclampsia, a pregnancy complication characterized by high blood pressure and signs of damage to another organ system.

- **Post-Surgery Recovery:** Bhramari is beneficial in the healing process post-surgery, aiding in quicker recovery and reduction of inflammation.

- **Alleviates Mental Stress:** This practice is particularly effective in relieving feelings of anger, anxiety, and stress, promoting a state of calm and relaxation.

- **Improves Sleep:** It's known for its ability to combat insomnia, helping expectant mothers find better rest and sleep quality.

- **Throat Health:** By gently vibrating the throat area, helps prevent throat diseases.

- **Controls High Blood Pressure:** Bhramari can be beneficial in managing high blood pressure, making it safer for both mother and baby.

- **Spiritual Relaxation:** On a spiritual level, this pranayama deepens relaxation and inner peace, enhancing spiritual awareness and connection.

Precautions for Bhramari Pranayama:

- **Positioning:** Avoid practicing Bhramari pranayama lying down. Sitting comfortably with a straight spine is recommended to ensure optimal breathing and safety.

- **Ear Infections:** If you have any ear infections, it's best to skip this practice to avoid exacerbating the condition.

- **Avoid Kumbhaka:** Do not hold your breath (Kumbhaka) during this pranayama. The focus should be on a continuous, smooth flow of breath.

How to Practice Bhramari Pranayama:

- Sit comfortably with your spine erect and your shoulders relaxed. You can sit on a chair or the floor with a cushion for support.

- Close your eyes and take a few deep breaths to center yourself.

- Place your index fingers on the cartilage between your cheeks and ears.

- Take a deep breath in, and as you exhale, gently press down on the cartilage while making a soft humming sound like a bee. The vibration should be felt in your head.

- Repeat this process for 4-5 cycles, focusing on the soothing sound and vibration with each exhalation.

4. Ujjayi breathing

Ujjayi Breathing, often referred to as "Ocean Breath" due to its distinctive sound resembling the gentle roll of ocean waves, is a beneficial pranayama technique, especially during pregnancy. This practice involves a specific way of breathing that not only enhances oxygenation but also fosters a deep sense of calm and focus. Here's how you can practice Ujjayi Breathing safely during pregnancy:

How to Practice Ujjayi Breathing:

Find a Comfortable Seat:

- Begin by sitting in a comfortable yoga pose that allows your spine to be straight and upright. You can sit on a cushion or a chair to ensure your comfort throughout the practice.

Close Your Mouth:

- Keep your mouth closed throughout the practice. Ujjayi Breathing is performed entirely through the nostrils, emphasizing control and the movement of air.

Inhale Deeply:

- Inhale deeply through your nose, filling your lungs with air. Focus on drawing the breath deeply into your belly and chest without straining.

Constrict Your Throat:

- As you exhale, gently constrict the back of your throat to create a soft hissing or ocean-like sound. This action is similar to fogging up a mirror, but with the mouth closed. The sound should be audible to you and help in focusing the mind and deepening the breath.

Maintain the Rhythm:

- Continue with this pattern of breathing, maintaining the rhythmic inhalation and the controlled, audible exhalation for several minutes. Aim for smooth, steady breaths that keep you relaxed and centered.

Benefits of Ujjayi Breathing During Pregnancy:

- **Enhanced Oxygenation:** By focusing on deep, controlled breaths, Ujjayi Breathing improves oxygen flow to both the mother and the baby.

- **Stress Reduction:** The calming effect of the ocean-like sound and the focused breathing technique help reduce stress levels and promote mental clarity.

- **Increased Focus and Presence:** Practicing Ujjayi encourages mindfulness, helping expectant mothers to stay present and connected with their bodies and babies.

- **Preparation for Labor:** The control and focus required for Ujjayi Breathing can be particularly beneficial during labor, aiding in pain management and relaxation.

Precautions:

While Ujjayi Breathing is generally safe during pregnancy, it's crucial to listen to your body and avoid any practices that cause discomfort or strain. Always practice under the guidance of a qualified instructor, especially if you are new to pranayama, and consult with your healthcare provider to ensure that it's appropriate for your specific situation.

*****

Pranayama, especially exercises focusing on exhaling, can significantly enhance the sense of relaxation and comfort for pregnant women. It's an accessible form of therapy that not only supports maternal well-being but also promotes fetal health by potentially improving placental circulation. Here's a simple guide to practicing an exhale-focused breathing technique that can be easily incorporated into your daily routine:

Steps for Exhale Breath Practice:

Find Your Seat:

Begin by sitting in a position that feels comfortable and stable. You can sit on a chair with your feet flat on the ground or a cushion on the floor with your legs crossed.

Hand Placement:

Gently place the palms of your hands on the sides of your ribcage. This tactile connection can help you become more aware of your breath and how your lungs expand and contract.

Relax Your Upper Body:

Allow your elbows to point outward naturally, and take a moment to relax your shoulders down away from your ears, reducing any tension in your upper body.

Inhale Deeply:

Take a deep breath in, focusing on filling your lungs so that you feel them expanding sideways under your hands. This helps maximize the breath's effectiveness.

Exhale Fully:

Gently exhale, releasing the breath out completely. Imagine any stress or tension leaving your body with this exhale.

Observe the Breath:

As you continue to breathe, notice the sensation of your lungs filling up on the inhale and contracting on the exhale. This awareness can enhance the relaxation benefits of the practice.

Maintain Deep, Relaxed Breathing:

Aim to take five to eight deep, yet relaxed breaths. Each cycle should feel soothing and not forced.

Additional Tips for Easier Breathing:

Good Posture: Whether you're sitting or standing, maintaining good posture can significantly improve your breathing efficiency. Keep your spine long and shoulders relaxed.

Sleeping Position: Prop yourself up during sleep to make breathing easier. Using pillows to support your upper body in a semi-sitting position can help reduce breathing discomfort, especially as your pregnancy progresses.

Meditation

Meditation during pregnancy is a powerful tool for nurturing both maternal and fetal well-being. The practice offers a peaceful retreat from the daily swirl of thoughts – often ranging between 12,000 to 60,000 a day, with 95% being repetitive. This mental chatter, largely focused on past and future events, can induce stress, elevating cortisol levels with potential negative impacts on the fetus.

Effect of Meditation During Pregnancy:

Emotional Connection: Meditation fosters a deep emotional bond between you and your baby, enhancing mutual well-being.

Stress Reduction: By lowering cortisol levels, meditation effectively reduces stress, creating a serene environment for both mother and child.

Insomnia Relief: It addresses sleep issues, helping expectant mothers enjoy more restful nights.

Mental Clarity: Meditation clears the mind, boosting creativity and readiness for both childbirth and parenting.

Prevents Postpartum Depression: Regular practice during pregnancy can decrease the likelihood of experiencing postpartum depression.

Fetal Protection: It contributes to reducing the risks associated with pre-term labor and Intrauterine Growth Restriction (I.U.G.R).

Scientific Insights on Meditation:

Physiological Benefits: Meditation has been shown to decrease oxygen consumption and heart rate, indicating a state of deep rest.

Skin Resistance: It significantly increases skin resistance (by up to 250-500% in Galvanic Skin Response), reflecting reduced stress levels.

Nervous System Activation: The practice revitalizes the nervous system, enhancing overall bodily functions.

Healing Capacity: Meditation can heal or mitigate psychosomatic and somatopsychic disorders, bridging the gap between mind and body health.

Stress and Anxiety Reduction: It effectively eliminates mental stress and anxiety, contributing to emotional stability.

Pain and Blood Pressure Management: Regular meditation can lessen headaches and manage hypertension, improving quality of life.

Lactic Acid Reduction: Just 15-30 minutes of meditation can lower lactic acid levels by 33%, alleviating muscle tension and fatigue.

Alpha Waves: The practice increases alpha brainwaves, associated with calmness, enhancing mental peace and happiness.

Pregnant mothers can significantly benefit from meditation by choosing themes or focuses that resonate with them personally. Here are several meditation subjects that can aid in creating a peaceful, positive pregnancy experience:

Meditation on the Rising Sun: Starting your day with meditation focused on the sunrise can fill you with energy, hope, and a sense of new beginnings.

ॐ **Sound:** Chanting or focusing on the sound "ॐ" (Om) helps in calming the mind, reducing stress, and connecting with the universe's vibrational energy.

Full Moon: Meditating on the image or energy of the full moon can bring a sense of calm, balance, and reflection, enhancing emotional well-being.

Prayer and Vedic Mantras: Reciting prayers or Vedic mantras during meditation can spiritually uplift and provide a sense of protection and blessings for both mother and baby.

Nature: Focusing on elements of nature, such as the sound of waves, rustling leaves, or a gentle breeze, can help ground you and foster a deep connection with the natural world.

Celebration Music: Listening to uplifting and joyous music during meditation can enhance feelings of happiness and celebration of the new life within.

Religious Gods and Goddesses: Meditating on figures from your religious or spiritual tradition can offer strength, guidance, and a sense of being cared for during your pregnancy journey.

Trataka: This practice involves focusing your gaze on a single point, such as a candle flame, to improve concentration and calm the mind.

Of Ideal Great Men, Ideal Thoughts: Reflecting on the lives and teachings of individuals you admire can inspire and motivate you, filling your meditation practice with positive, aspirational energy.

Incorporating exercise, yoga, dhyan (meditation), and pranayama (controlled breathing) into your pregnancy journey offers a holistic approach to maintaining both physical and mental well-being. Here's a summary of how each practice contributes to a healthier pregnancy:

Exercise During Pregnancy

Regular physical activity is essential for staying healthy and comfortable throughout pregnancy. It can help maintain your fitness level, support better sleep, reduce pregnancy discomforts like back pain, and potentially make labor easier.

Yoga for Expectant Mothers

Yoga offers a gentle way to stay active. Its focus on stretching, strength, and balance is ideal for adapting to your changing body. The controlled movements and breathing also aid in stress reduction and promote a state of relaxation, helping you connect with your baby on a deeper level.

The Role of Dhyan (Meditation)

Meditation provides a peaceful retreat for the mind, helping to ease anxiety and stress associated with pregnancy. It encourages a mindful awareness of your body and baby, enhancing emotional bonds and assisting in navigating pregnancy's physical and emotional shifts with grace.

Pranayama (Controlled Breathing)

Pranayama practices are especially beneficial during pregnancy, offering ways to improve lung capacity, enhance blood circulation, and bring about a profound sense of calm. Techniques such as deep abdominal breathing and Nadi Shodhan (alternate nostril breathing) can be particularly helpful in managing morning sickness, fatigue, and other common pregnancy symptoms.

Incorporating These Practices

Blending exercise, yoga, meditation, and pranayama into your prenatal care regimen can significantly boost your and your baby's health and well-being. These practices not only prepare your body for childbirth but also nurture your mental and emotional health, providing a balanced approach to pregnancy care.

Consultation with Healthcare Professionals

Before starting on any new exercise program or yoga practice during pregnancy, it's crucial to consult with a healthcare provider. They can offer personalized advice based on your health status, pregnancy progress, and any potential risks, ensuring that your routine is safe and beneficial for you and your unborn child.

This holistic approach to pregnancy care, physical activity, mental relaxation, and emotional connection, sets the foundation for a healthy, joyful pregnancy journey, ultimately fostering a positive environment for both mother and child.

A Note

Remember, your pregnancy journey is unique, and so is your way of finding balance and joy during this special time. Listening to your body and giving yourself permission to rest when needed is just as important as staying active. Accept these practices with kindness towards yourself, knowing that by caring for your emotional well-being, you're also creating a nurturing environment for your baby to thrive.

As you move and breathe with intention, you're not just preparing your body for childbirth;

you're also nurturing your heart and mind, building a foundation of strength, calm, and resilience that will support you through pregnancy and into motherhood.

*"A new baby is like the beginning of
all things—wonder, hope, a
dream of possibilities."*
– Eda J. Le Shan

Action Item

Incorporate a gentle prenatal yoga routine or a daily walk into your schedule. Aim for at least 20 minutes of physical activity that makes you feel good.

Chapter 6

"Nurturing Life: The Essential Guide to Healthy Eating During Pregnancy"

Nourishing Body and Soul

Nourishing your body and soul during pregnancy is about much more than just eating healthy foods. It's about finding a balance that looks after every part of you. What you eat not only feeds your body but also affects how you feel emotionally and spiritually. Taking care of yourself in this way is not just about the nutrients on your plate but also about the love and attention you give to your body and the little life growing inside of you.

Eating well during pregnancy sets up a strong foundation for your health and your baby's growth. But it's also deeply linked to your journey into motherhood, shaping how you connect with and prepare for bringing a new life into the world. Here, we'll talk about why good nutrition matters and how it can help make delivery smoother. We'll also share tips on planning your meals to fit your pregnancy needs, how to eat mindfully to satisfy your body's signals without going overboard, and which superfoods are especially good for you and your baby.

Understanding the importance of nutrition during pregnancy is crucial because the food you consume is the main source of nutrients for your growing baby. A balanced diet ensures that both you and your baby receive the necessary vitamins, minerals, and nutrients for optimal health, growth, and development.

Why Nutrition is Key:

- **Fetal Development:** Essential nutrients like folic acid, iron, calcium, and omega-3 fatty acids play significant roles in the development of the baby's brain, skeleton, and vital organs. Folic acid, for instance, is critical in preventing neural tube defects.

- **Maternal Health:** Adequate nutrition supports the mother's health, helping to manage pregnancy symptoms and reducing the risk of pregnancy-related conditions such as anemia, gestational diabetes, and preeclampsia.

- **Energy Requirements:** During pregnancy, the body's energy needs increase. A balanced diet provides the extra calories needed for the baby's growth, especially in the second and third trimesters.

- **Healthy Weight Gain:** Gaining a healthy amount of weight during pregnancy is important for the baby's health and can make it easier for the mother to return to her pre-pregnancy weight post-delivery.

- **Emotional Well-being:** Nutrition also impacts the mother's emotional well-being. A diet rich in omega-3 fatty acids, for example, can lower the risk of postpartum depression.

When considering what to eat during pregnancy, it's important to balance nourishing foods with avoiding those that might pose risks. Here's a closer look at some specific foods and their effects:

Papaya: It's generally advised to avoid unripe papaya as it can potentially harm the pregnancy. Unripe papaya contains latex, which may lead to uterine contractions.

Seeds: Some seeds should be avoided due to their potential effects on hormone levels and pregnancy.

Ripe Papaya: Eating a slice or two of ripe papaya can be beneficial due to its vitamin content, but it's best to consume in moderation.

Mango: Rich in vitamins and minerals, a slice or two of mango can contribute positively to your pregnancy diet, offering nutritional benefits.

Pineapple: While there's a common belief that pineapple should be avoided due to its bromelain content, eating a few slices occasionally, especially when in season, is generally considered safe. Avoid the core, as it contains higher concentrations of bromelain.

Seasonal Fruits: In general, seasonal fruits are a great addition to a pregnancy diet. They provide essential vitamins and minerals that support the health of both mother and baby.

The diet of a pregnant woman should support the physical, mental, and emotional development of the child within the womb. Beyond just physical health, the emotional and mental state of the mother can profoundly affect the baby. A child's health is intricately linked to the mother's physical, mental, and emotional wellbeing.

While much focus is often placed on the physical and external aspects of health during pregnancy, it's crucial not to overlook the importance of mental, emotional, and even spiritual health. A balanced diet that includes a variety of nutrient-rich foods can help support all these aspects, contributing to a healthier pregnancy and a strong foundation for the baby's growth and development.

Why specific diet important for pregnant women?

Understanding the significance of a specific diet for pregnant women is crucial for ensuring the health and well-being of both the mother and her developing baby. Modern science supports the idea that a nutritious diet plays a key role in maintaining the mother's health and significantly contributes to the child's physical development.

During pregnancy, the body requires additional energy and nutrients to support the growing fetus. This is not just about physical strength; the mental and emotional readiness of the mother also plays an essential role, especially during delivery. A well-balanced diet ensures that the mother has the stamina, excitement, and positive mental and emotional state needed for a smooth delivery process.

Post-delivery, a healthy diet continues to be crucial. The nutrients consumed by the mother are passed to the baby through breast milk, which is the baby's primary source of nourishment in the early stages of life. Breast milk's composition, rich in essential nutrients, supports the infant's growth and immune system development.

Moreover, a nutritious diet during pregnancy can help prevent complications at the time of delivery. It reduces the risk of conditions such as gestational diabetes, high blood pressure, and pre-eclampsia, all of which can affect the health of both mother and baby.

How a Balanced Diet Supports Both Mother and Baby:

A balanced diet during pregnancy includes a variety of fruits, vegetables, whole grains, lean proteins, and healthy fats. Each food group provides specific nutrients that are key to health:

- **Fruits and Vegetables:** Rich in vitamins, minerals, and fiber, they support digestive health and reduce the risk of pregnancy constipation.

- **Whole Grains:** Provide essential carbohydrates, fiber, and B vitamins, helping to meet the mother's increased calorie needs and support fetal development.

- **Lean Proteins:** Important for the growth of fetal tissue, including the brain, and helps the mother's body increase its blood supply.

- **Dairy or Fortified Alternatives:** Source of calcium and vitamin D, crucial for the development of the baby's bones and teeth.

- **Healthy Fats:** Sources like avocados, nuts, and seeds, along with omega-3 fatty acids from fish or supplements, support brain development.

Stay Hydrated

- **Water:** Drinking plenty of water is essential. It helps transport nutrients to your baby, aids in digestion, and reduces the risk of urinary tract infections.

- **Hydrating Foods:** Include foods with high water content like cucumbers, strawberries, and watermelon in your diet. They're refreshing and add to your daily fluid intake.

Listening to Your Body

- **Mindful Eating:** Pay attention to your hunger and fullness signals. Pregnancy is not about eating for two in terms of quantity but rather ensuring you're getting double the nutrient quality.

- **Cravings and Moderation:** While it's okay to indulge in cravings occasionally, focus on nutrient-dense foods that contribute to your and your baby's health. Find healthier alternatives to satisfy those cravings.

Practical Tips for Meal Planning

- **Batch Cooking:** Prepare and freeze meals in advance. This can be particularly helpful in the later stages of pregnancy when energy levels might be lower.

- **Snack Wisely:** Keep healthy snacks like nuts, yogurt, or fruit handy. They can provide a quick nutrient boost without the added sugars and fats of processed snacks.

- **Hydration Reminder:** Set reminders to drink water throughout the day. Keeping a water bottle with you can also encourage regular sips.

Adjustments and Considerations

- **Supplements:** Consult with your healthcare provider about any necessary supplements like folic acid or iron, to ensure you're getting all the necessary nutrients.

- **Dietary Restrictions:** For special dietary needs or restrictions, consider consulting a nutritionist to tailor a plan that ensures you're meeting your pregnancy nutrition goals.

Food Converts In To Fluid After The Digestion Process.

According to Ayurveda, as detailed by Charak, the food we consume undergoes a transformation process after digestion. It's believed that the essence of food is converted into fluid, which then nourishes the body. This philosophy emphasizes the importance of the six tastes in Ayurveda, each playing a unique role in our health and well-being, especially during pregnancy. These tastes include:

Madhur (Sweet): Foods that are sweet in taste are not just about sugar; they also include grains, dairy, and fruits. They are vital for building the tissues of the body and provide energy. During pregnancy, sweet foods can help in the healthy growth of the fetus and ensure that the mother maintains her energy levels.

Bhawan (Salty): Salty tastes, found in foods like salt and seaweed, help maintain the electrolyte balance in the body. In moderation, salt is essential for hydration and proper cell function. However, excessive salt intake during pregnancy should be avoided as it can lead to water retention and high blood pressure.

Ambh (Tangy): Tangy or sour foods, such as citrus fruits and fermented products, can stimulate digestion and enhance appetite. They also provide a good source of vitamin C, crucial for both the mother's and baby's immune systems.

Katu (Bitter): Bitter foods like leafy greens and herbs help detoxify the body and support liver function. Including bitter tastes in a pregnancy diet can aid in preventing nausea and boosting the digestive process.

Tikha (Spicy): While overly spicy foods may need to be moderated during pregnancy to avoid discomfort, mildly spicy foods can improve digestion and metabolism. Spices like ginger and turmeric are beneficial in small quantities.

Kashay (Astringent): Astringent foods, including legumes and raw fruits and vegetables, can aid in absorbing excess water and tighten tissues. They also contribute to a balanced diet by providing fiber, which helps prevent constipation during pregnancy.

Eating for two

"Eating for two" is a phrase often heard during pregnancy, but it's more about the quality of nutrition than the quantity. The food choices you make during pregnancy have a profound impact on your health, your baby's development, and the overall experience of pregnancy and delivery. Understanding this impact can help guide you towards making nutritional choices that benefit both you and your baby.

Nutrition's Role in Pregnancy

Nutrition during pregnancy does more than just fuel your body; it lays the groundwork for your baby's health. Every bite you take can contribute to your baby's growth and development, affecting everything from brain development to bone strength. For instance, omega-3 fatty acids are crucial for brain development, while calcium supports bone growth.

The Myth of Eating for Two

While you might need more calories during pregnancy, the increase is not as significant as the phrase "eating for two" implies. In fact, during the first trimester, you might not need extra calories at all. It's during the second and third trimesters that your calorie needs increase, and even then, it's only by about 300-500 calories a day. This is roughly the equivalent of a snack or small meal.

Quality Over Quantity

The emphasis should be on nutrient-dense foods that provide the vitamins, minerals, and other nutrients your body needs to support a healthy pregnancy. This includes a variety of fruits, vegetables, whole grains, lean proteins, and healthy fats. These foods offer the building blocks for your baby's growth and help manage pregnancy symptoms and energy levels.

Impact on Delivery

Good nutrition can also influence the delivery process. Women who maintain a balanced diet are less likely to experience complications such as gestational diabetes or preeclampsia, which can impact delivery. Furthermore, a well-nourished body is better prepared for the physical demands of labor and recovery after birth.

Three acts:

In the journey towards motherhood, nutrition plays a crucial threefold role: nourishing the mother, supporting the child's development, and preparing the body for milk production. Understanding these aspects can greatly enhance both maternal and fetal health during and after pregnancy.

Nutrients for the Mother: A healthy diet before delivery is vital. It ensures the birth of a healthy baby, typically weighing between 2.5 to 3.5 kg. During pregnancy, the uterus expands up to five times its normal size, from around 30 gm to 15 times more, eventually increasing 500 times to accommodate the growing fetus. A nutritious diet supports this remarkable transformation, fuels the development of the breasts for future milk production, and strengthens the womb, the nurturing space where the child grows. Moreover, a well-balanced diet can prevent common pregnancy issues like indigestion.

Development of the Child: The nutrients a mother consumes directly impact the fetal growth and development. Starting from a small yolk sac, which initially nourishes the embryo, the child's sustenance depends entirely on the mother's diet, facilitating growth from a few cells to a 2.5 to 3 kg newborn.

Milk Production Process: Post-delivery, the mother's body initiates the milk production process to continue providing essential nutrients to the newborn. A healthy diet during pregnancy sets the stage for a successful and abundant milk production, ensuring the baby continues to receive the nutrients needed for healthy development outside the womb.

Neglecting a healthy diet can lead to several adverse outcomes, including the risk of diseases for the child, complications in achieving pregnancy, miscarriage, preterm delivery, excessive bleeding, thyroid issues, and neural tube defects, among others. The mother's health and the child's development could be severely compromised.

The Importance of Early Check-ups: Seeking medical guidance before the third month of pregnancy is crucial. Doctors often recommend supplements like folic acid and zinc, which are essential for preventing birth defects and ensuring healthy fetal development. A balanced diet—consuming the right foods in the right amounts—is essential. However, nutrition is just one piece of the puzzle. A healthy pregnancy also depends on an effective daily routine and a positive mental and emotional environment. These elements combined create the ideal conditions for both the mother and the child during this critical period.

Preconception Preparations

Pre-conceptional preparations are vital steps taken even before the start of pregnancy, aimed at ensuring the best health outcomes for both the mother and the child. This phase is often riddled with numerous questions concerning diet, such as "what to eat," "when to eat," "what not to eat," and "how much to eat." The plethora of advice available, ranging from medical science to Ayurveda to various scriptures, can often be confusing. To navigate this, let's delve into an integrated approach that combines the wisdom of medical science, Ayurveda, and scriptures.

The Journey of Diet:

Since when:

The preparation for a healthy pregnancy begins much before conception. It's advised to start focusing on your health from day one, and even before you plan to become pregnant. This ensures that your body is in the best possible condition to support a new life.

What to eat:

- Modern science emphasizes a balanced diet consumed at proper times. It highlights the importance of both basic nutrients required for maintaining good health and additional nutrients needed specifically for pregnancy.

- Ayurveda, on the other hand, advises on including foods that balance the doshas (body energies) and promote physical, mental, and emotional well-being.

- Scriptures advocate for food that is virtuous and cultured. This means consuming foods that are not only physically nourishing but also positively affect your mind and spirit.

The moral of integrating medical science, Ayurveda, and scriptural wisdom is to acknowledge that pregnancy nutrition is multifaceted. It's not just about eating a balanced diet; it's also about consuming food that nurtures the body, mind, and soul. The focus should be on:

- Ensuring the diet is balanced and timely, as recommended by modern science, to meet the physical nutritional needs.

- Incorporating Ayurvedic principles to balance the body's energies and promote overall well-being.

- Choosing foods that are virtuous and cultured, as guided by scriptures, to positively impact the emotional and spiritual health of both the mother and the developing baby.

Why Not To Eat

Navigating nutrition during pregnancy involves not just knowing what to eat but also understanding what to avoid to ensure both the mother and the developing baby receive optimal nourishment.

Ayurveda and modern dietary science together provide a comprehensive guide on maintaining a balanced diet that supports the intricate processes of pregnancy.

What Not to Eat?

Ayurveda emphasizes the importance of avoiding foods that could disrupt the body's balance. This includes highly processed foods, those high in refined sugars, and excessive intake of cold and raw foods which might be harder to digest.

Ayurvedic Monthly Routines suggest a dynamic approach to nutrition, tailoring dietary needs as the pregnancy progresses, ensuring a balance of basic and additional nutritional elements like proteins, carbohydrates, fats, minerals, micronutrients, and antioxidants. The ideal ratio for a balanced diet is 4:4:1, encompassing these components to support the development of nerves, bones, skin, blood, and arteries.

Daily Water Intake should be between 10-12 glasses to support the body's increased demands during pregnancy.

Protein is crucial for the development of the baby's physical structures and should be sourced from milk, yogurt, lentils, and a mix of flours. A recommended mix is 7 kg wheat, 1 kg legumes, and

1 kg soybean, washed, dried, and finely ground. This blend offers a rich source of protein.

Carbohydrates serve as the primary energy source. Unpolished rice and minimally washed vegetables like potatoes help preserve carbohydrates.

Fats should be consumed in moderation, about 5 teaspoons per day, focusing on unsaturated fats that don't form blockages in arteries. Traditional cow ghee, mustard oil, olive oil, canola oil, sunflower oil, and groundnut oil are recommended for their beneficial effects during pregnancy.

Vitamins, Minerals, Micronutrients, and Antioxidants play a significant role in enhancing the body's immunity. A mix of 10 gm ripe groundnut, 15 gm legumes, and 25 gm green gram beans can significantly increase the intake of these essential nutrients, bolstering the body's defenses against the harmful effects of chemicals. This mix also supports digestion, skin health, blood formation, hair health, vision, heart health, brain function, and cholesterol management.

ORS - Original, Regional & Seasonal foods like various seasonal fruits and green vegetables should be prioritized to ensure the intake of fresh, nutrient-rich produce that aligns with the body's natural needs.

Additional Nutrients might be required due to personal dietary preferences, lifestyle changes, or specific nutritional deficits. While a balanced diet rich in various vegetables, including green ones, can generally meet these needs, some situations may necessitate supplementing with vitamins, minerals, and other nutrients.

Understanding and applying these dietary principles during pregnancy can help ensure that both the mother and baby are nourished, setting a strong foundation for health and well-being.

Key dietary pillars during pregnancy:

During pregnancy, nutrition takes on a critical role, not just in supporting the health of the mother but also in ensuring the optimal development of the baby. Understanding the four essential pillars of diet during this period can significantly influence the outcome of pregnancy and the health of both mother and child.

First Quarter (First Three Months): Brain Nutrients + Brain Development

The initial three months focus on consuming nutrients essential for the baby's brain development. Sources of DHA like almonds, walnuts, flaxseed, and soya cottage cheese are vital. Choline can be found in groundnuts and dairy products, while iodine is abundant in milk, flour, bananas, and spinach. Folic acid is crucial during this period and is found in green vegetables, legumes, and beans. Other important nutrients include B12, found in soya milk and dairy, and zinc, present in green vegetables and legumes. Omega 3, necessary for brain development, can be sourced from green leafy vegetables, walnuts, and mustard oil.

Second Quarter (Another Three Months): Growth Nutrients + Physical Development

The focus shifts to the physical development of the baby, requiring a balanced intake of protein, carbohydrates, and fats. Calcium and magnesium, found in dairy products and almonds respectively, support bone development. Vitamin D from sunlight and dairy helps absorb calcium efficiently, while iron from green leafy vegetables ensures healthy blood development.

All 9 Months: Immune Nutrients + Immunity Development and Digesting Nutrients (Healthy Energy)

Throughout the pregnancy, it's important to consume foods that boost the immune system and aid digestion. Vitamin C from citrus fruits, vitamin E from vegetables like carrots and tomatoes, and fructo-oligosaccharides from bananas and wheat support immunity and digestive health. Additionally, thiamine (vitamin B1) is crucial for energy production from food, found in sunflower seeds and black lentils.

Preparing Soybean Tofu

Soybean tofu is a nutritious addition to the pregnancy diet. To make it, soak soybeans, remove the peels, and create a paste. Boil the paste, stirring to prevent sticking, then filter. Curdle the soya milk with lemon or yogurt, filter to separate the paneer (cottage cheese), and use the remaining paste in dishes like flatbreads.

All Quarters: Hydration and Fiber

Water and fiber are essential throughout pregnancy to manage constipation and support overall health. Multigrain flour, unpolished rice, and fresh fruits (not juice) contribute to a balanced diet that supports the mother's and baby's health.

Water

Water plays an essential role during pregnancy, with increased needs compared to non-pregnant individuals. Approximately 4-6 liters of water daily is beneficial for expecting mothers. It's important to start the day by consuming three glasses of water in the morning and continue to drink 10-12 glasses throughout the day.

Why is water so crucial during pregnancy? Here are several reasons:

- It helps reduce constipation by aiding the digestive process.

- It facilitates the removal of waste products from the body through sweat and urine.

- It helps regulate the body's temperature, keeping both the mother and baby comfortable.

- Drinking water boosts energy and willpower, essential during pregnancy.

- It keeps the skin soft and hydrated, reducing discomfort from skin stretching.

Masaru Emoto, a Japanese scientist, conducted research that suggested water could carry more than just physical benefits. He proposed that treating water with positive intentions, such as holding a glass of water between the hands and drinking it with a sense of reverence, can enhance its benefits, making it as beneficial as nectar.

To maximize the benefits of water during pregnancy, it's advised to:

- Drink water slowly and in a seated position to ensure proper absorption and digestion.

- Limit water intake during meals to only what is necessary to avoid diluting digestive enzymes.

- Consume water ideally one hour before or 1-1.5 hours after meals to support optimal digestion.

- Remember that water is the essence of life, supporting the well-being of both the mother and the developing baby throughout pregnancy.

Gut-Brain Connection

The connection between our gut and brain, often referred to as the "Gut-Brain Connection," plays a crucial role in how our emotions and intelligence are influenced by our diet. This fascinating relationship is studied in nutritional psychiatry, a branch of advanced nutritional neuroscience that examines the effects of diet on our mental health.

Here's why our diet has such a powerful impact on our mood and mental well-being:

Two Brains in One Body: We have a brain in our head and another in our gut. The gut is often called the "second brain" because it produces about 95% of serotonin, a neurotransmitter that makes us feel good. This means a healthy gut can lead to a happier mood.

Good Bacteria Equals Good Mood: Beneficial bacteria in our gut help us absorb nutrients better, which in turn helps produce more serotonin. This positive feedback loop between good bacteria and brain function means a healthier diet can lead to a better mood.

The Impact of Diet on Mental Health: Diets high in refined sugars and processed foods are linked to depression, whereas a diet rich in vegetables, fruits, and unprocessed grains can boost energy and improve mood. Lisa Kilgour, a nutritionist, explains that a low level of neurotransmitters in the brain can lead to depression, while similar imbalances in the gut can cause digestive issues like constipation and slow digestion.

Diet's Role in Brain Size and Intelligence: Consuming a lot of junk food can negatively affect the hippocampus and lower IQ, as noted by researcher Felica Jack.

The ancient scriptures, including the Chandogya Upanishad, emphasise the importance of pure food for purifying the mind and soul, leading to liberation and enlightenment. According to Ayurveda and ancient wisdom, our diet should not only be physically nourishing but also pure, affecting our emotional and mental health. Pure (Satvik) foods, which are tasty, health-oriented, and good for the heart and mind, include vegetarian foods like lentils, whole grains, seasonal fruits, milk, yogurt, vegetables, and honey. Such a diet fosters qualities like patience, peace, forgiveness, and concentration, promoting physical health and emotional well-being.

Consultation Is Key

Consulting with a healthcare provider or a registered dietitian is crucial during pregnancy because every woman's body, every pregnancy, and every baby is unique. These professionals can offer personalized guidance that takes into account your health history, lifestyle, any pre-existing conditions, and specific nutritional needs. Here's why this personalized advice is so important:

Firstly, a healthcare provider can assess your overall health and any potential pregnancy complications that could affect your nutritional needs. For instance, if you're at risk for gestational diabetes, they might recommend a diet lower in simple sugars. Or, if you're carrying twins, they could suggest increasing your protein intake to support the growth of both babies.

A registered dietitian specialises in understanding the intricate balance of nutrients needed to support both you and your developing baby. They can provide detailed advice on how to incorporate essential nutrients into your diet, suggest meal plans, and even offer strategies for managing common pregnancy symptoms through diet, like nausea or constipation.

Personalised advice is particularly beneficial because it can adapt as your pregnancy progresses. Nutritional needs change from the first trimester through to the third, and postpartum too. A professional can guide you through these changes, ensuring you and your baby are supported at every stage.

Akbar and Birbal

The story of Akbar, Birbal, and the goat offers a profound insight into the delicate balance between nutrition and emotional well-being, particularly during the transformative period of pregnancy. It unfolds with Emperor Akbar presenting Birbal, his wisest advisor, with a challenge that at first glance seems straightforward yet is laced with complexity: to maintain a goat's weight precisely as it is over the course of a month, despite ensuring the animal is well-fed.

Birbal, known for his wit and intelligence, accepts the challenge without hesitation. He takes the goat under his care, providing it with an abundance of food to ensure it receives all the nutrients it needs. Under Birbal's watchful eye, the goat enjoys a diet rich and varied, aimed at promoting its health and vitality. One might expect that with such generous feeding, the goat would naturally gain weight.

However, Birbal had a unique strategy up his sleeve. Each night, after the goat had its fill, Birbal would place it near a lion's cage. The mere presence of the predator, the king of the jungle, instilled a deep sense of fear in the goat. This fear triggered a physiological response, increasing the goat's metabolism and causing it to burn calories at a rate that counteracted the weight it might have gained from its daily feasts.

When the month concluded and the goat was presented to Akbar, the emperor was baffled to find that, indeed, its weight had not changed. Curious and somewhat incredulous, Akbar demanded an explanation. Birbal then revealed his method, illustrating how the emotional state of fear had a direct impact on the goat's physical condition, preventing any change in its weight despite the abundant nourishment it received.

Just like the goat in the story, which remained the same weight due to the stress of fear, even when well-fed, pregnant women may find that stress and negative emotions can undermine the positive aspects of a nutritious diet.

During pregnancy, the importance of physical nutrition cannot be overstated, yet the story reminds us that emotional well-being holds equal weight. Stress, fear, and anxiety are not just feelings; they manifest physically, potentially leading to an increased heart rate, elevated blood pressure, and they might even impact the developing baby.

In the story where the goat faced the lion, it shows us something important for pregnant women too. When you're expecting, it's like having your own lions of worry. You might wonder if your baby is growing right, if everything is okay with their health, if your blood pressure is fine, or if the baby's weight is on track. These worries are like that lion standing in front of the goat, making it hard for you to get all the good from the healthy food and water you're taking in.

Even though eating healthy is super important for both you and your baby, stress and fear can stop you from getting all the benefits of this good nutrition. It's like the goat that couldn't put on weight because it was scared every night. If you're stressed, it can affect your baby's growth and your own health.

That's why being calm and happy every day when you're pregnant is so key. It helps your body use all the good stuff from your food and drink better, helping your baby grow strong and healthy.

How can you stay calm and happy? Recognising your worries is the first step. Then, try things that make you feel peaceful, like yoga for pregnant women, taking some quiet time to breathe and relax, or just doing things that make you smile. Talking to your doctor about your worries can help too. Knowing more about pregnancy and what's happening can make those worries seem smaller.

Eating right and staying hydrated are very important when you're pregnant, but so is keeping those worries – those lions – in check. Finding ways to stay peaceful and happy doesn't just help you feel better; it makes sure your baby gets the best start, too.

> *"A mother's arms are more comforting*
> *than anyone else's."*
> *– Princess Diana*

Action Item

Plan and prepare a week's worth of healthy, balanced meals. Include plenty of fruits, vegetables, whole grains, and lean proteins. Try to include one new nutritious recipe each week.

Chapter 7

"Nurturing Dreams: The Power of Sleep in Pregnancy"

The Power of Sleep

During pregnancy, your body goes through a lot of changes, and sleep is one area that's majorly affected. Hormones play a big part in this. As your body works to support your growing baby, hormonal changes can shake up your usual sleep patterns and even the quality of your rest.

For starters, the hormone progesterone goes up a lot during pregnancy. While progesterone is super important for keeping your pregnancy healthy, it also makes you feel more tired during the day. At night, though, it can make it harder to find a comfortable sleep position or stay asleep.

Then there's the fact that your body is working overtime to support your baby. This extra work can make you feel tired but, ironically, can also keep you awake. Plus, as your baby grows, you might find it harder to get comfortable in bed, leading to more tossing and turning.

Another thing is that pregnant folks often have to get up more during the night to go to the bathroom. This is because the growing uterus puts pressure on the bladder, making those middle-of-the-night bathroom trips more frequent.

All these changes can make it tough to get a good night's sleep, but rest is super important during pregnancy. Good sleep helps keep you and your baby healthy. It can boost your mood, make you feel less stressed, and give your body the energy it needs to take care of your growing baby.

During pregnancy, getting a good night's sleep can sometimes feel like a challenge. You might find yourself getting up often at night, dealing with an upset stomach or heartburn, feeling lower back pain, or experiencing leg cramps. Plus, as your body changes to make room for your baby, it can be tough to find a cozy way to lie down. These issues can make it hard to get the restful sleep you need.

Finding a comfy sleeping position is key to improving your sleep quality during pregnancy. Most experts suggest sleeping on your side, especially on your left side, as it increases the amount of blood and nutrients that reach your baby. This position can also help reduce swelling in your legs.

Using pillows can make a big difference, too. Placing a pillow between your knees or under your belly can provide extra support and help ease back pain or discomfort. Some people find pregnancy pillows, which are specially designed for this purpose, to be very helpful.

Avoiding certain positions is also important. Sleeping flat on your back after the first trimester is usually not recommended, as it can put pressure on a major vein that carries blood back to your heart from your lower body. This can reduce blood flow to your baby and cause backaches, digestive problems, and low blood pressure for you.

Getting comfortable and finding the right sleep position can take some experimenting, but it's worth it for you and your baby's health. With a few adjustments and the right support, you can improve your chances of getting the restful sleep you need during this special time.

How Hormones Affect Sleep

Progesterone Increase: Early in pregnancy, levels of progesterone rise sharply, which can contribute to increased daytime sleepiness and a desire for more naps. Despite making you feel sleepier, high progesterone levels can also disrupt your nighttime sleep, making it less restful.

Physical Changes: As pregnancy progresses, physical discomforts like back pain, heartburn, and the frequent need to urinate can interrupt sleep. The growing belly can make it hard to find a comfortable sleeping position.

Emotional Fluctuations: Emotional changes and anxiety about becoming a parent or the delivery can also impact sleep, making it harder to fall or stay asleep.

Sleep isn't just a time-out from the day; it's a critical part of ensuring both you and your baby are as healthy as possible during pregnancy. The link between getting enough sleep and the well-being of both mother and baby is stronger than you might think. Let's dive into why this restful period is so crucial.

When you get a good night's sleep, your body gets a chance to repair itself. This downtime is when your body does a lot of important work, like growing muscle, repairing tissue, and producing the hormones that your body needs to function properly. For a pregnant person, this repair time is even more critical because it supports the body in adapting to the changes and demands of pregnancy.

Adequate sleep also plays a significant role in regulating your emotions. We all know how a bad night's sleep can leave us feeling irritable or stressed the next day. During pregnancy, when your hormones are already doing a delicate dance, ensuring you get enough rest can help keep mood swings at bay and reduce stress levels. Lower stress levels are not just good for you; they're also beneficial for your baby. Stress has been linked to various pregnancy complications, so keeping it in check is key.

Good sleep has been connected to a healthier pregnancy outcome. It can reduce the risk of developing certain complications like gestational diabetes and high blood pressure, both of which can affect the health of you and your baby. Adequate rest can also contribute to the proper growth and development of your baby in the womb.

Sleep deprivation can have the opposite effect, increasing the risk of complications and affecting your immune system. When you're well-rested, your body's defenses are better equipped to fight off infections, which is especially important during pregnancy when your immune system is naturally a bit suppressed to accommodate your growing baby.

Good sleep during pregnancy can set the stage for a smoother delivery. Being well-rested can give you the energy you need to face the physical demands of labor and delivery. And after the baby arrives, having established good sleep habits can help you navigate the challenging postpartum period when sleep can be even more fragmented.

Giving Body and Mind Rest

Getting enough sleep during pregnancy isn't just about feeling rested; it's a fundamental aspect of your health and well-being, as well as your baby's. Let's break down why sleep is so vital during this unique time in your life.

Sleep does more than just recharge your batteries. It plays a critical role in supporting the various changes and demands your body experiences during pregnancy. Here's how it helps:

Supports Physical Health: Your body is doing the incredible work of growing another human being. This process requires a lot of energy and can put a strain on your body. Sleep gives your body the chance to rest and repair, ensuring you and your baby's physical health is supported. For example, during deep sleep, your body can focus on growing muscle tissue, repairing cells, and balancing hormones—essential tasks for a healthy pregnancy.

Boosts Emotional Well-being: It's common to experience a wide range of emotions during pregnancy, from joy and anticipation to anxiety and fear. A good night's sleep can help manage these emotions, reducing stress and anxiety levels. When you're well-rested, you're more likely to have a positive outlook, which is beneficial not just for you but also for your baby. Studies have shown that reduced stress and anxiety can lead to healthier pregnancy outcomes.

Enhances Brain Function: Pregnancy can sometimes feel like it's accompanied by a case of "baby brain," where you might be more forgetful or find it hard to concentrate. Adequate sleep can help combat this by improving cognitive functions like memory, attention, and decision-making. Getting enough rest can help you feel more mentally sharp and capable of handling the tasks and decisions that come with pregnancy.

Strengthens the Immune System: Your immune system naturally undergoes changes during pregnancy to protect the growing fetus. This can sometimes leave you more susceptible to infections. Sufficient sleep helps bolster your immune system, making it easier for your body to fight off illnesses. This is crucial for preventing infections that could affect your pregnancy.

Prepares for Labor and Delivery: As your due date approaches, having a reserve of energy becomes increasingly important. Quality sleep in the weeks leading up to delivery can ensure you're physically and mentally prepared for the labor process. While the connection between rest and an easier delivery isn't guaranteed, being in a better state of health can certainly contribute to a smoother experience.

Quality Rest

Quality rest plays a significant role in ensuring a healthier pregnancy journey and can even contribute to a potentially easier delivery. This isn't just about catching up on sleep but understanding how deep, restorative sleep affects both your body and your baby in profound ways.

Well-rested bodies can manage the physical demands of pregnancy better. This means that your body is more prepared for the marathon that is labor and delivery. Think of it as training for a big event; you wouldn't want to go into it tired and unprepared. Sleep is your body's way of training and building up the strength you'll need.

Quality sleep has been linked to reduced stress levels. High stress can increase the risk of complications during delivery, such as prolonged labor. When you're well-rested, your body's stress hormones are lower, making it easier for your body to function as it should during labor. It's like going into delivery with a clearer mind and a body that's ready to focus on the task at hand.

Sleep also impacts your emotional well-being, which is incredibly important during delivery. When you're more relaxed and less anxious, you're able to cope with the demands of labor more effectively. This positive emotional state can make the delivery experience more manageable and even more positive. It's about setting a calm, strong foundation for one of the most significant moments of your life.

Quality rest isn't just a luxury; it's a crucial part of preparing your body and mind for the journey of pregnancy and the process of delivery.

Best sleeping position During Pregnancy

Finding the most comfortable and healthy sleeping position is crucial during pregnancy. As your belly grows, lying on your left side with your knees slightly bent is often recommended. This position isn't just about comfort; it significantly benefits blood circulation for both you and your baby.

In the early stages of pregnancy, sleeping on your stomach is okay, but as you enter the second trimester, it's best to avoid this position due to your growing belly.

Sleeping on your left side is particularly beneficial because it enhances blood flow. This ensures that essential nutrients and oxygen efficiently reach your baby and vital organs. It can also help reduce swelling in your legs and ankles, a common concern for many pregnant individuals.

While sleeping on your right side might put unnecessary pressure on your liver, it's generally safe to do so for brief periods. The key is to find a sleeping arrangement that keeps you comfortable and supports healthy blood flow. Using pillows for extra support around your belly or between your knees can make side-sleeping more comfortable and effective.

Sleep position to avoid

While sleeping on your right side for short periods is generally okay, it's important to avoid certain sleeping positions during the later stages of pregnancy, especially stomach sleeping and lying on your back.

As your pregnancy advances, lying on your back can cause the weight of your growing uterus to press on major blood vessels like the aorta and the vena cava. This pressure can make it more challenging for your heart to pump blood efficiently to you and your baby. You might even feel discomfort or dizziness when you wake up.

Back sleeping can also increase pressure on your spine, potentially leading to or worsening lower back pain—a common issue during pregnancy. Plus, it's linked to a higher likelihood of snoring and experiencing other sleep-related breathing problems.

While advice often suggests avoiding back sleeping from the 20th week of pregnancy, recent research indicates that back and right side sleeping during the first 30 weeks may not significantly increase the risk of stillbirth. Reflecting on this, some health experts now recommend that pregnant individuals choose the most comfortable sleeping position for them during the first two trimesters.

Here are some simple strategies to enhance your sleep comfort during pregnancy:

Bend Your Knees: Side sleeping with your knees slightly bent can offer back support. This position can make sleeping more comfortable.

Use Pillows for Support: Placing a pillow between your legs, behind your lower back, or under your belly can reduce discomfort. Consider trying a full-body pillow designed for pregnant individuals for added support.

Choose a Comfortable Mattress or Topper: A mattress or topper that alleviates pressure points, like those made from egg crate foam, can help ease hip pain associated with side sleeping.

Elevate Your Upper Body: If heartburn disturbs your sleep, try elevating the head of your mattress or bed. Sleeping in a slightly upright position can help manage heartburn symptoms.

Sleep on the Left Side of the Bed: Positioning yourself on the left side of the bed might encourage you to maintain sleeping on your left side, promoting better blood flow.

One Survey Was Conducted For Sleep Analysis

In a study focused on understanding sleep during pregnancy, it was recommended that adults, including those who are pregnant, should aim for 7 to 9 hours of sleep each night. Despite this, pregnant individuals often experience less sleep, increased wakefulness, and more daytime sleepiness compared to those who aren't pregnant. About 80% of pregnant women report poor sleep quality throughout their pregnancy.

This lack of quality sleep is linked to several negative outcomes for both the mother and baby, such as preeclampsia, gestational diabetes, the need for cesarean deliveries, and preterm births. It can also lead to tiredness, fatigue, and problems with thinking and concentration. Given these risks, there's a clear need for safe, non-medical ways to improve sleep during pregnancy, as using medication to aid sleep can pose safety concerns.

Exercise emerges as a safe, effective way to manage poor sleep, not just for those who aren't pregnant but also for pregnant individuals. Exercise encompasses a variety of activities, including leisurely, transportation, caregiving activities, and more structured forms of exercise. The mental benefits of exercise, along with its physical restorative effects, contribute to better sleep. Additionally, getting sunlight during outdoor exercise can help regulate the body's natural sleep-wake cycle, enhancing sleep quality.

The health benefits of exercising during pregnancy are well-documented, including a lower risk of gestational diabetes, preeclampsia, and less likelihood of needing interventions like cesarean sections during childbirth. However, research shows that many pregnant women do not get enough exercise. Various factors, from physical symptoms to psychosocial barriers, can prevent them from exercising adequately.

Attitudes and beliefs about exercise play a crucial role in whether pregnant women engage in physical activity. Similarly, positive attitudes towards sleep are linked to better sleep duration and quality. While evidence suggests that exercise can improve sleep in pregnant women, there's still much to learn about their attitudes and beliefs toward using exercise as a means to enhance sleep.

Sleep Strategies for Each Trimester

First Trimester

The first trimester brings about a lot of changes, and among these are new sleep patterns and managing fatigue. As your body begins the incredible process of growing a new life, it also kicks into high gear hormonally, which can have a big impact on how you sleep. Let's explore some strategies to navigate these changes and ensure you're getting the rest you need during these initial months of pregnancy.

Adapting to New Sleep Patterns: It's common to feel more tired than usual during the first trimester. Your body is producing higher levels of progesterone, a hormone essential for maintaining pregnancy that also has a sedative effect. You might find yourself needing more sleep or feeling drowsy at times of the day when you used to feel wide awake. Listening to your body is key. If you feel tired, allow yourself short naps or go to bed earlier. However, try to keep a consistent sleep schedule as much as possible to regulate your sleep patterns.

Managing Fatigue: The fatigue you experience in the first trimester can be quite profound. It's your body's way of telling you to slow down and allow it to direct energy towards supporting the developing embryo. To manage this, prioritize rest whenever you can. Break down tasks into smaller, manageable chunks, and don't hesitate to ask for help when you need it. Light exercise, like walking or prenatal yoga, can also help boost your energy levels and improve sleep quality, as long as your healthcare provider gives you the green light.

Creating a Comfortable Sleep Environment: Your usual sleeping position might not feel as comfortable now. Experiment with different positions to find what works best for you. Although it's early in pregnancy, starting to sleep on your side, particularly your left side, can increase the amount of blood and nutrients that reach your baby. Use pillows to support your body and create a comfortable sleeping position.

Mind Your Diet: What you eat and drink can significantly impact your sleep quality. Try to maintain a balanced diet and avoid large meals, caffeine, and sugary snacks close to bedtime. Opt for light, nutritious snacks if you're hungry before bed. Staying hydrated is important, but try to limit fluids a couple of hours before bedtime to minimize nighttime trips to the bathroom.

Relaxation Techniques: Incorporating relaxation techniques into your bedtime routine can help you wind down and prepare for sleep. Techniques like deep breathing, gentle stretching, or listening to calming music can signal to your body that it's time to rest. Establishing a bedtime routine that includes these practices can make falling asleep easier.

Second Trimester

The second trimester often brings a welcome change in how you feel, including improvements in sleep. Sometimes called the "honeymoon period" of pregnancy, many of the challenges of the first trimester, like nausea and extreme fatigue, start to ease up, and yet the physical discomforts of the third trimester haven't begun. This is a great time to focus on maximizing the quality of your sleep.

Enjoying More Comfortable Sleep: As your body adjusts to being pregnant, you might find it easier to get comfortable at night during the second trimester. The increase in abdominal size is usually still manageable, allowing for a variety of sleeping positions. Continuing to sleep on your side, especially the left side, is beneficial as it promotes optimal blood flow to your baby. Using pregnancy pillows can also help support your growing belly and keep you comfortable throughout the night.

Maintaining a Sleep Schedule: With the easing of first-trimester symptoms, you can focus on maintaining a regular sleep schedule. Going to bed and waking up at the same time each day can help regulate your body's sleep-wake cycle, leading to better sleep quality.

Taking Advantage of Energy Levels: The second trimester often comes with a boost in energy. Use this to your advantage by incorporating moderate exercise into your routine, which can improve sleep. Activities like swimming, prenatal yoga, or walking can be especially beneficial. Just be sure to finish any vigorous activity a few hours before bedtime to give your body time to wind down.

Mindful Eating for Better Sleep: Continue to eat a balanced diet and pay attention to how what you eat affects your sleep. Try to avoid heavy or large meals close to bedtime, and limit your intake of caffeine and sugary foods. Snacking on small, protein-rich foods before bed can help stave off hunger and stabilize blood sugar levels through the night.

Relaxation Before Bed: Establishing a relaxing bedtime routine remains important during the second trimester. Activities that soothe the mind and body, such as reading, taking a warm bath, or gentle stretching, can prepare you for a restful night.

Third Trimester

The third trimester marks a period of rapid growth and final preparations before your baby arrives. As your body changes and your baby grows, you might find sleep becomes more elusive due to increased physical discomfort and anticipation of the birth. However, there are ways to manage these challenges and even use this time to prepare for postpartum sleep habits.

Managing Discomfort for Better Sleep: As your belly grows, finding a comfortable sleeping position becomes more challenging. Continuing to sleep on your side, particularly your left side, can help improve circulation to your baby and relieve pressure on your back. Use pregnancy pillows or regular pillows to support your belly, back, and between your knees to ease discomfort and keep your spine aligned.

Practice Good Sleep Hygiene: Maintaining a consistent sleep schedule becomes even more crucial. Establish a relaxing nighttime routine that signals to your body it's time to wind down. This might include activities like reading, taking a warm bath or gentle stretching exercises specifically designed for pregnancy.

Prepare for Frequent Nighttime Awakenings: The need for frequent bathroom trips and baby movements can interrupt your sleep. Keep the path to the bathroom clear and use a soft nightlight to minimize the disruption caused by these awakenings. Though it might be tempting, try to avoid looking at your phone or other screens during these wakeups, as the blue light can make it harder to fall back asleep.

Nap Wisely: If you're experiencing fatigue, short daytime naps can help. However, limit naps to 20-30 minutes earlier in the day to avoid disrupting your nighttime sleep.

Anticipate and Plan for Newborn Sleep Patterns: The third trimester is a good time to start thinking about how you'll manage sleep once your baby arrives. Newborns have very different sleep needs and patterns, often waking every few hours to eat. Familiarize yourself with safe sleep practices for infants and consider strategies for sharing nighttime duties with your partner or support system.

Focus on Relaxation Techniques: Techniques that promote relaxation and stress relief can be particularly helpful in the third trimester. Practices like mindfulness, deep breathing, or prenatal yoga can ease anxiety and improve sleep quality. These techniques can also be valuable after your baby is born, helping you cope with the stress and demands of new parenthood.

Communication and Support: Talk with your healthcare provider about any sleep difficulties you're experiencing. They can offer specific advice or interventions to help manage discomfort and improve sleep. Additionally, discuss your postpartum plan with your partner or support system to ensure you have the help and support you need once the baby arrives.

Tips For Better Sleep

Maintain a Regular Sleep Schedule: Going to bed and waking up at the same time every day can help regulate your body's internal clock and improve the quality of your sleep.

Create a Sleep-Inducing Environment: Make your bedroom conducive to sleep by removing bright lights and reducing noise. Keep electronic devices, like phones and computers, out of the bedroom to avoid distractions.

Nap Smartly: If you're feeling extra tired, short naps during the day can help. Try to keep them brief (20-30 minutes) and avoid napping late in the day to not disrupt your nighttime sleep.

Practice Relaxation Techniques: Stress can interfere with sleep, so incorporate relaxation exercises into your routine. Techniques like deep breathing, meditation, or gentle yoga can help calm your mind and prepare your body for rest.

Watch Your Evening Intake: Try to minimize eating large meals or consuming foods and drinks that can disrupt sleep, such as those high in sugar or caffeine, in the evening.

Limit Caffeine: Reducing caffeine intake, especially in the hours leading up to bedtime, can help prevent sleep disturbances.

Consider Prenatal Vitamins: Taking prenatal vitamins that include iron and folic acid not only supports your baby's development but may also reduce symptoms of restless legs syndrome, which can affect sleep.

Keep Moving: Regular, moderate exercise can improve sleep quality. Stretching and strengthening exercises are particularly good for reducing back pain and leg cramps, common pregnancy discomforts.

Consult Your Doctor: If you're struggling to sleep well or think you might have a sleep disorder, it's important to talk to your healthcare provider. Conditions like obstructive sleep apnea, heartburn, or restless legs syndrome can affect sleep quality and have implications for your pregnancy.

By incorporating these tips into your daily routine, you can improve your sleep quality during pregnancy, *benefiting both you and your baby.*

Action Item

Develop a relaxing bedtime routine that includes activities like reading a book, taking a warm bath, or practicing deep breathing exercises to help you unwind and prepare for restful sleep.

Chapter 8

"Nurturing Transformation: Embracing Change and Growth in Pregnancy"

Embracing Change and Growth

Pregnancy is a journey that's about more than just your body changing to make room for a new life. It's a time when you grow a lot as a person. You see changes in how you think, how you feel about yourself, and how you connect with others. It's a chance to see things in a new way, to learn, and to get ready for the big changes that come with being a mom.

When you look at pregnancy as a chance to grow, you start to see all the new experiences and challenges as opportunities. It's not just about your baby getting bigger inside you; it's about you growing on the inside too. This journey teaches you so much about yourself, helps you connect more deeply with your own feelings, and prepares you for the new job of being a mom.

Being open to all the changes during pregnancy can make this time even more special. It helps you to be kind to yourself, to pay attention to what your body and heart are telling you, and to find strength in all the new things you're going through. Remember, each day is a step closer to meeting your baby and starting a new part of your life, filled with new discoveries, strengths, and a deeper sense of love and connection.

Another significant sign to watch for is if you miss your period. This is usually the most noticeable and earliest indicator that you might be pregnant. So, if you've missed a period following unprotected intimacy, it might be time to consider taking a pregnancy test. However, keep in mind that there are other reasons you might miss a period, such as stress, very intense exercise, or not eating the right nutrients, which can all disrupt your hormonal balance.

If you're thinking about when the right time is to take a pregnancy test, it's generally as soon as you've missed a period. Home pregnancy tests work by detecting a hormone called human chorionic gonadotropin (hCG) in your urine. Around 10-15 days after you've missed your period, these tests can usually tell if you're pregnant.

If you take a test and it comes back positive, the next step is to visit your healthcare provider. They can do a blood test and an ultrasound to officially confirm your pregnancy.

As you go through your pregnancy journey, each week might bring a new set of experiences and symptoms. These could range from sleepless nights and headaches to feeling nauseous, developing stretch marks, experiencing mood shifts, disliking certain foods suddenly, and even cramps. There's also something called implantation bleeding, which is a bit of light spotting or bleeding that can happen about ten days after conception. But if you notice that you're bleeding a lot, it's crucial to get in touch with a doctor right away because heavy bleeding could indicate a miscarriage. The chance of losing a pregnancy is usually higher in the first three months and can be due to various reasons, including ectopic pregnancy, molar pregnancy, or what's known as a chemical pregnancy. While these situations are relatively uncommon, it's important to be aware of them.

After the first trimester, the likelihood of a miscarriage significantly decreases. Despite this, you might still face other challenges as your pregnancy progresses. Growing belly, frequent trips to the bathroom, discomfort in your body, stress, heartburn, and acne can all be part of the pregnancy experience.

Adopting a healthy lifestyle, eating a balanced diet, taking prenatal vitamins, and keeping up with regular doctor's visits can help you manage these issues. Using a pregnancy pillow for support under your belly or between your legs can make sleeping or resting more comfortable. Sleeping on your left side is also recommended.

Getting a pregnancy massage can be wonderfully relieving for muscle and joint pains associated with pregnancy, and it's also great for lowering stress and boosting circulation. Just be sure the massage therapist is skilled in prenatal techniques. However, massages are generally advised against during the first trimester or if your pregnancy is considered high-risk. Always consult your doctor before going for a massage.

Pregnancy brings a mix of emotions and changes, some expected and others surprising. Building resilience during this time means finding ways to handle these changes with strength and flexibility. Here are simple strategies to help you adapt and stay strong:

Learn as much as you can: Knowing what to expect during pregnancy can make changes less daunting. Read up or chat with healthcare providers to get a clear picture.

Lean on others: Having people to talk to, like family, friends, or folks going through similar experiences, can offer comfort and advice when you need it.

Keep calm: Techniques like deep breathing or gentle yoga can help keep stress levels down and make it easier to deal with surprises.

Be open to change: Plans might shift, and that's alright. Being open to going with the flow can make unexpected changes easier to manage.

Control what you can: Focus on the things you can influence, like eating well, getting enough sleep, and staying active. It gives a sense of control amid uncertainty.

Continuous Improvement (CANI)

Continuous and Never-Ending Improvement, or CANI, is all about always getting better. For someone going through pregnancy, this idea is especially important. Pregnancy is a time when everything is changing—how you look, how you feel, and even how you think. By using the CANI approach, you can face these changes positively and keep growing.

During pregnancy, CANI means finding little ways every day to improve your health, your surroundings, and how you connect with people close to you. Maybe one day, you learn a new fact about taking care of babies, another day you might try a new healthy snack, or spend some extra time talking about the future with your partner.

Improvement doesn't need to be a big thing. Even small steps, done regularly, can make a big difference over time. The best part about CANI during pregnancy is that it helps you get ready for your new baby and helps you keep learning and growing as a family.

So, think of your pregnancy as a chance to keep getting better in small ways. This mindset not only helps you prepare for your baby but also starts a habit of always learning and growing that can benefit your whole family.

Applying CANI to Pregnancy

Applying the idea of Continuous and Never-Ending Improvement (CANI) to pregnancy involves taking small, daily steps towards better health, preparing for delivery, and learning about parenting. Here's how you can do it:

Health Improvement: Start with simple changes to your diet, like adding more fruits and vegetables or drinking more water. Regular gentle exercise, like walking or prenatal yoga, can also help. Consider mindfulness or relaxation techniques to manage stress. Small improvements each day can lead to significant health benefits over time.

Preparation for Delivery: Educate yourself about the birthing process. Attend prenatal classes, read books, or watch educational videos. Practicing relaxation and breathing techniques can also prepare you for labor. Preparing a birth plan is another step towards feeling more in control and ready for the big day.

Learning About Parenting: Start by reading articles or books on parenting, or join a parenting group online where you can learn from others' experiences. Learning how to care for a newborn, understanding their sleep patterns, and knowing the basics of feeding (breastfeeding or bottle-feeding) can be done gradually during pregnancy.

Pregnancy In Each Trimester

Pregnancy unfolds in stages, offering a remarkable journey that varies from one woman to another. It's often broken down into three trimesters, with each one marking a distinct phase of growth and changes for both the mother and the developing baby.

First Trimester (Weeks 1–12): This initial phase is crucial as it lays the foundation for the baby's development. Early on, the fusion of sperm and egg forms what will become the fetus, and the body starts to adjust hormonally to support this new life. Symptoms like morning sickness and fatigue are common, but they signify that your body is preparing for the journey ahead. By the end of the first trimester, the fetus has a heartbeat, and foundational structures for organs, limbs, and bones are established. It's a time of rapid and critical development.

Second Trimester (Weeks 13–27): Often considered the most comfortable phase, the second trimester is when many of the more challenging early symptoms might fade. The baby grows larger and stronger; you can start to feel movements as the baby kicks and stretches. This period allows for more detailed ultrasounds, where you can see clearer images of your baby, and for many, find out the sex if they choose. It's a time when the bond between mother and baby strengthens, as the physical presence of the baby becomes more apparent.

Third Trimester (Weeks 28–40): The final stretch is a period of growth and preparation. The baby's movements become stronger, and the body prepares for birth. It's a time to learn about labor and delivery, to make final preparations for the baby's arrival, and to monitor your health closely. The baby is getting ready for life outside the womb, practicing breathing, and gaining the fat needed to regulate body temperature after birth.

Each trimester brings its own set of challenges and milestones. Listening to your body, getting regular check-ups, and preparing mentally and emotionally for childbirth are key. As the due date approaches, anticipation grows, but it's important to remember that the timing of delivery can vary. Whether it's at 37 weeks or beyond 40 weeks, the goal is a healthy baby and mother.

Family Health Habits

Building healthy habits as a family truly changes the game. It's about turning what could be fleeting moments of health consciousness into a steady stream of choices that enrich your family's life every day. Think of it as weaving wellness into every aspect of your daily routine, so it becomes second nature, a part of who you are as a family unit.

In this journey, every family member plays a crucial role, and together, you create a circle of health that ripples out, influencing not just your own lives but also the community around you. It's a way of living that brings you closer, strengthens your bonds, and sets a foundation for a lifetime of health and happiness. This is the power of building healthy habits as a family—it's life-changing.

Shared Meals, Shared Moments: Sitting down together for meals isn't just about eating; it's a chance to connect, to share your day's highs and lows, and to listen to each other. It's these moments that can turn a simple meal into a cherished family memory, reinforcing the idea that being together matters just as much as the nutritional value of what's on the plate.

Movement as a Bonding Activity: Encouraging each other to stay active, whether through walks after dinner, weekend bike rides, or playful competitions in the backyard, shows that caring for our bodies is also a way to care for our relationships. It's about finding joy in movement and sharing that joy with the ones you love.

Conscious Screen Time: In today's world, screens are everywhere, making it easy to get lost in digital spaces. Setting boundaries around this, for both kids and adults, isn't about restriction but about making space for other meaningful activities that can enrich your lives in ways screens can't.

Snack Smarter, Together: Choosing healthy snacks is a small change that can have a big impact. It's a way to show that taking care of your body doesn't have to be complicated or restrictive but can be enjoyable and delicious. Plus, experimenting with new, healthy snacks can be a fun adventure in itself.

Stay Hydrated, Stay Happy: Something as simple as drinking enough water can become a shared goal that encourages everyone to look after themselves and each other. It's about creating habits that feel good and do good, fostering a sense of well-being that radiates through the family.

Rest: Recognizing the importance of rest, and modeling that for your children, teaches them that it's okay to take a step back, to recharge, and to listen to their bodies. Creating a peaceful bedtime routine can become a cherished part of the day, a time for quiet connection and reflection.

Open Hearts and Minds: Creating an environment where feelings are openly discussed, and challenges are met with support, sets a powerful example. It says that it's okay to be vulnerable, to ask for help, and to talk about what's on your mind. This openness can strengthen the emotional health of the family, creating a safe space for everyone.

Learn and Grow Together: Whether it's trying out a new recipe, starting a family project, or learning a new skill together, these experiences can strengthen bonds, create memories, and encourage a love of learning that extends beyond the home.

This journey is rich with opportunities for connection, learning, and growth, touching every aspect of life.

Action Item

Reflect on the changes happening in your body and life by keeping a pregnancy journal. Write about your experiences, emotions, and the growth you notice in yourself and your baby.

Chapter 9

Cesarean vs. Vaginal Birth

Choosing between a natural delivery (ND) and a Cesarean section (LSCS) often leads to many questions and concerns among expectant parents. While this book provides extensive guidance on cultivating habits that support a normal delivery, it's crucial to understand that there are no guarantees in childbirth. Each pregnancy and delivery is unique, and various factors can influence the outcome.

Adopting the principle from the Bhagavad Gita about doing one's duty efficiently and with good faith is helpful here. This perspective encourages you to focus on preparing for the birth through healthy practices, while also being open to the outcomes, whatever they may be. The primary aim is to ensure the health and safety of both mother and baby, whether that results in a natural delivery or a Cesarean section.

Many expectant parents wonder about the right time to choose one type of delivery over the other. Common questions include inquiries about the possibility of a normal delivery after having one or more Cesarean sections. To address these concerns, it's essential to understand the birth process in detail and to have open, informed discussions with your healthcare provider.

Trust between a patient and their doctor is foundational. Taking the time to gather information, attending consultations, and discussing your particular medical history and needs with your doctor are all crucial steps. These discussions should help you feel comfortable and informed about your choices.

There are several obstetric, medical, and surgical conditions that might necessitate a Cesarean section to ensure the safety and health of both mother and baby. Some of these conditions include but are not limited to:

- Prolonged labor that does not progress

- Baby's position being unsuitable for vaginal birth (e.g., breech position)

- The mother having health issues like high blood pressure or diabetes that could pose risks during vaginal delivery

- Previous Cesarean sections, depending on the incisions and uterus condition

- Signs of distress in the baby during labour

- Placental issues such as placenta previa or placental abruption

Understanding these factors and having a trusted healthcare provider can guide you through making the best decision for both you and your baby. Remember, the goal is a healthy delivery for mother and child, whether that means a vaginal birth or a Cesarean section.

Cesarean Section

Cesarean sections, commonly referred to as C-sections, are sometimes necessary to ensure the safety and health of both the mother and the baby during childbirth. The decision to proceed with a C-section can depend on various medical conditions and circumstances, categorized into absolute and relative indications.

Absolute Indications for Cesarean Section:

Absolute indications for a Cesarean section leave no room for choice; the procedure is imperative to prevent potential risks to both mother and child. These include:

- **Contracted Pelvis:** A pelvis where the conjugate diameter at the brim is less than 7 cm or where other dimensions of the pelvis are too small to allow a vaginal delivery.

- **Obstruction in the Pelvic Canal:** This can be caused by a fibroid tumor, an ovarian cyst, or a tumor of the sacrum, which physically blocks the passage that the baby must travel through during birth.

- **Exceptionally Large Fetus:** Sometimes referred to as fetal macrosomia, where the baby is significantly larger than average, particularly if the baby's head does not engage and the anterior parietal eminence is noticeably beyond the symphysis pubis.

- **Multiple Previous C-sections:** Having had two or more C-sections in the past can increase the risk of complications like uterine rupture during vaginal birth.

- **Transverse Lie:** This is a situation where the baby is positioned side-to-side within the uterus, which can complicate the natural process of childbirth.

- **Placenta Previa:** A condition where the placenta covers part or all of the cervix, making vaginal delivery impossible without risking severe bleeding.

In cases like these, a Cesarean section is the only option to ensure the safe delivery of the baby and the well-being of the mother.

Relative Indications for Cesarean Section:

Relative indications suggest that while a vaginal delivery could be possible, a Cesarean section may present a safer or more viable alternative for various reasons. These can include:

- **Prolonged Labor:** When labor does not progress normally, possibly due to the baby's position or a slowdown in cervical dilation.

- **Signs of Fetal Distress:** Such as abnormal heart rates, which might indicate the baby is not handling labor well.

- **Medical Conditions in the Mother:** Such as hypertension or diabetes, where a quick delivery might become necessary to avoid complications.

- **Herpes Infection:** Active genital herpes infection at the time of labor, which could be transmitted to the baby during a vaginal birth.

- **HIV/AIDS:** When a mother has HIV/AIDS, a C-section might be recommended to reduce the risk of transmitting the virus to the baby.

Choosing between a vaginal delivery and a Cesarean section often depends on multiple factors, including the mother's health, the baby's condition, and specific risks associated with childbirth. Expectant mothers must discuss their particular situation with healthcare providers to make informed decisions that align with the best possible outcomes for their health and their baby's well-being.

Cesarean vs. Vaginal Birth

When considering how to welcome your baby into the world, it's essential to weigh the options between a vaginal birth and a cesarean section (C-section). Each method has its advantages and potential risks, and the right choice often depends on various personal and medical factors.

Deciding on a Cesarean Section

A C-section is a surgical procedure used to deliver a baby through incisions in the abdomen and uterus. It's often recommended under certain conditions to ensure the safety of both mother and baby:

- **Multiples:** If you are expecting twins, triplets, or more, the positioning and health of the babies may necessitate a C-section.

- **Breech Position:** If your baby is not in the head-down position and instead positioned bottom-first or feet-first, a C-section might be safer.

- **Previous C-sections:** If you have had a previous C-section, especially with a vertical incision, your doctor might recommend this route again to avoid risks like uterine rupture.

- **Medical Conditions:** Certain health issues such as diabetes, high blood pressure, or active genital herpes can make vaginal birth risky, making a C-section a safer alternative.

- **Placenta Previa:** This condition occurs when the placenta covers the cervix, obstructing the baby's exit during birth. It typically necessitates a C-section to prevent complications like severe bleeding.

Situations That May Lead to a Cesarean During Labor

Even if you plan for a vaginal birth, circumstances during labor can change, leading to the decision for a C-section. These might include:

- **Labor not progressing:** Sometimes, labor stalls or the cervix stops dilating, which can prolong labor and put the baby at risk.

- **Signs of distress in the baby:** If monitoring shows that the baby is in distress, such as abnormal heart rates or other signs of being under stress, a C-section allows for quicker delivery to safeguard the baby's health.

- **Cord prolapse:** This rare but urgent complication occurs when the umbilical cord slips through the cervix into the vagina before the baby does, which can compress the cord and reduce the baby's oxygen supply.

- **Uterine rupture:** This is a rare tearing of the uterus that can endanger both mother and baby.

Deciding whether to opt for a vaginal birth or a C-section involves careful consideration of your health, your baby's condition, your previous medical or birth history, and the current circumstances of your labor. It's crucial to have open discussions with your healthcare provider, who can offer guidance based on your specific health scenario and the wellbeing of your baby.

Vaginal Birth

Opting for a vaginal birth is often considered the default choice for many expectant mothers, and for good reason. It generally presents fewer risks than a cesarean section (C-section) and can provide a quicker recovery time. Here are several benefits of choosing a vaginal birth:

Health Benefits of Vaginal Birth

- **Lower Risk of Complications:** Women who deliver vaginally tend to have fewer complications such as severe bleeding, which might require a blood transfusion.

- **Reduced Risk of Infections:** The chance of developing a postpartum infection, such as a uterine infection, is lower with vaginal births. These infections can be serious enough to warrant a return to the hospital in the weeks following childbirth.

- **Less Internal Scarring:** Vaginal births minimize the risk of internal scarring in the uterus. Such scarring can lead to future reproductive issues, including complications with placental placement, ectopic pregnancies, and potential infertility.

- **Fewer Surgical Risks:** Unlike C-sections, vaginal births avoid the risks associated with major abdominal surgery, such as bladder or intestinal injuries.

Potential Challenges with Vaginal Birth

While vaginal births are generally safer, they are not without their challenges:

- **Pelvic Floor Damage:** One potential downside is the strain on a mother's pelvic floor muscles, which can lead to long-term issues with bladder and bowel control. These problems may require surgical intervention later in life.

- **Birth Trauma:** The use of instruments like forceps or vacuums, prolonged pushing, or a large baby can increase the risk of trauma during delivery. An episiotomy, which is a surgical cut made at the opening of the vagina during childbirth, can also contribute to this risk.

Despite these potential challenges, the American College of Obstetricians and Gynecologists continues to support vaginal births as a safer alternative to C-sections for most women, given the overall lower risk profile.

Making the Decision

It's crucial to discuss all your options with your healthcare provider. They can offer personalized advice based on your health history, the progression of your pregnancy, and any potential risks to you and your baby. By understanding both the benefits and risks associated with vaginal birth, you can make an informed decision that aligns with your personal health needs and birth preferences.

Pros and Cons

When it comes to choosing between a vaginal delivery and a cesarean section (C-section), each method comes with its own set of advantages and drawbacks:

Vaginal Delivery Advantages:

- Usually involves a shorter recovery period for the mother compared to a C-section.

- There's a lower chance of suffering from infections and significant blood loss.

- Natural labor and delivery trigger the release of hormones that promote mother-baby bonding and can make breastfeeding easier.

Vaginal Delivery Disadvantages:

- There's a possibility of vaginal tears or the need for an episiotomy, which is a cut made at the vaginal opening to help deliver the baby.

- Labor can be prolonged and physically exhausting.

- There is a risk of damaging the pelvic floor muscles, which can lead to long-term issues like incontinence or organ prolapse.

Caesarean Section Advantages:

- Delivery can be planned, which helps in organizing medical care and personal arrangements.

- Avoids the risks associated with pelvic floor damage, which are more common in vaginal deliveries.

- Sometimes a C-section is the safer option for certain health conditions or pregnancy complications.

Caesarean Section Disadvantages:

- Recovery time after a C-section is typically longer and may involve more discomfort and restrictions.

- Increased risk of surgical complications such as infections, blood clots, and accidental injury to organs.

- Each subsequent C-section can pose more risks, potentially limiting the number of safe pregnancies a woman can have.

Ultimately, choosing between a vaginal delivery and a cesarean section depends on several factors, including the health of the mother and baby, personal preferences, and the guidance of healthcare providers. It's crucial to have detailed discussions with your medical team to make a well-informed decision that best suits your situation.

In Many Conditions, We Can Give Trial Of Labour

1. In certain circumstances, a trial of labor after cesarean (TOLAC) may be considered. This approach allows women who have previously undergone a cesarean section to attempt a vaginal delivery. However, TOLAC is only recommended under specific conditions to ensure safety:

2. The surgical scar from the previous C-section must be thoroughly healed.

- The mother should be closely monitored for any signs of complications such as uterine rupture.

- There should be immediate availability of surgical intervention if the need for a repeat cesarean arises.

Healthcare providers typically use various assessment tools, such as the Flamm VBAC score, to evaluate the suitability of a trial of labor. This helps in determining the likelihood of a successful vaginal birth after cesarean, ensuring that both mother and baby remain safe throughout the process.

3. When it comes to twin pregnancies, the decision between a vaginal birth and a cesarean section can depend on several factors including the positions of the fetuses and the comfort level of the delivering obstetrician with managing twin births. If both fetuses are positioned favorably, and the mother attempts labor, there's a relatively high chance of a vaginal delivery—about 65% to 75%. The likelihood of a combined vaginal delivery and cesarean delivery (for one of the twins) ranges from about 3% to 10%.

However, with an experienced obstetrician who is skilled in the active management of twin deliveries during the second stage of labor, the likelihood of a successful vaginal delivery can increase to as high as 85%. Despite planning for a vaginal delivery, you might choose to have an elective cesarean section, or your healthcare provider might recommend one if potential complications arise. Additionally, even if a vaginal birth is planned, circumstances during labor such as changes in the babies' conditions or lack of progress in labor might necessitate an emergency cesarean section.

4. When discussing breech deliveries, it's important to understand the positioning of the baby as the due date approaches. Approximately 3-4% of babies remain in a breech position by the time a pregnancy reaches full term. The likelihood of a breech position decreases as the pregnancy progresses: early on, around 22-25% of babies are in a breech position before the 28th week. This percentage drops to about 7-15% by the 32nd week. By full term, most babies have moved into the head-down position necessary for a typical vaginal delivery.

    A breech position means the baby is positioned to deliver feet or buttocks first rather than the head, which can complicate the delivery process. Managing a breech delivery often involves specific considerations and preparations:

- **Monitoring:** Continuous monitoring of the baby's position during the later stages of pregnancy is crucial to identify a breech position early.

- **Decision Making:** Depending on factors like the baby's size, the mother's health, and the baby's exact position, healthcare providers might suggest attempting to turn the baby into the correct position through an external cephalic version (ECV) or planning for a breech delivery.

- **Delivery Options:** Some breech babies can be delivered safely through vaginal delivery, especially if the healthcare provider is experienced in breech births. However, a planned cesarean section is often recommended for breech babies to reduce risks associated with breech vaginal deliveries.

- **Personalized Care:** Each case is unique, and decisions about how to handle a breech pregnancy should be made in consultation with healthcare providers, considering all the available information about the mother and baby's health.

- Several factors can increase the likelihood of a baby being in a breech position, which means the baby might be positioned with feet or buttocks aimed to come out first rather than the head. These factors include:

- **Prematurity:** Babies born before 37 weeks are more likely to be breech.

- **Uterine anomalies or fibroids:** Irregularities in the shape or size of the uterus can prevent the baby from turning into the head-down position.

- **Polyhydramnios:** Excessive amniotic fluid can allow too much movement of the baby, including into breech positions.

- **Placenta previa:** When the placenta covers the cervix, it can inhibit the baby's ability to turn head-down.

- **Fetal abnormalities:** Certain conditions like central nervous system malformations, neck masses, or chromosomal abnormalities can prevent normal positioning.

- **First pregnancy:** In first pregnancies, the uterine muscles are typically more rigid, which can affect how the baby is positioned.

While most babies turn head-down by 37 weeks of pregnancy, some may not shift into this position until just before birth. If a baby remains in a breech position, vaginal delivery can be challenging or even risky. The American College of Obstetricians and Gynecologists (ACOG) recommends considering an external cephalic version (ECV) between 36 and 38 weeks. This procedure involves physically manipulating the baby into a head-down position from outside the mother's abdomen and is performed in a hospital setting by trained medical staff. However, success rates for ECV are about 50%, and it's not without risks.

Potential complications from attempting a vaginal breech delivery can be severe and include:

- **Trauma:** Issues like extended arms or head during delivery.

- **Placental abruption:** The placenta may detach prematurely.

- **Injury to abdominal organs:** Pressure or trauma during delivery can damage the baby's organs.

- **Broken fetal neck:** An extremely rare but possible injury if delivery is mismanaged.

- **Umbilical cord prolapse:** This can cut off the baby's oxygen supply leading to asphyxia.

Due to these risks, expectant mothers with a breech baby must discuss all options with their healthcare provider to make the safest choice for delivery.

So For Happy Delivery

For a positive delivery experience, it's important to follow several key steps:

- **Follow all recommended habits:** Stick to the health and wellness routines advised during pregnancy to prepare your body and mind for delivery.

- **Trust your doctor:** Have faith in the expertise of your healthcare provider. They have the experience and knowledge to guide you through the delivery process.

- **Bring a support person:** Whether it's your husband, a relative, or a close friend, having someone you trust by your side can provide comfort and support during labor and delivery.

- **Let the doctor do their best:** Allow your healthcare provider to make the necessary decisions during delivery. They are trained to handle various situations that may arise.

- **Avoid questioning every decision:** While it's important to understand the process, constantly questioning your doctor's decisions with doubt can be counterproductive.

- Trust that they are making the best choices for your health and the health of your baby.

- **Be patient:** Wait for your doctor to make informed decisions about the need for a cesarean section. Doctors typically resort to a C-section only when it's absolutely necessary for the safety of the mother and baby.

Remember, medical professionals aim to ensure the safest possible outcome for both you and your baby. They do not take unnecessary risks that could compromise their care and reputation.

"Every child begins the world anew."
– Henry David Thoreau

Action Item

Educate yourself about both birth options by attending a childbirth education class or reading reliable resources. Make a list of questions to discuss with your healthcare provider to make an informed decision.

Chapter 10

Accepting Your Journey into Parenthood

Preparing for parenthood is an exciting and transformative experience that profoundly impacts new mothers. This period of adaptation involves significant physical, emotional, and hormonal changes. While much attention is rightly given to the health and well-being of the newborn, it's equally important to focus on the mother's needs during this time.

After pregnancy, mothers require thorough and ongoing care to recover and adjust healthily. The postpartum period is not just about healing physically but also about managing the emotional transitions associated with motherhood. Ensuring comprehensive healthcare during this time supports mothers in adapting to their new roles, helping them nurture their babies while also taking care of their own well-being. This care is crucial for the mother to regain strength and stability, enabling her to provide the best care for her newborn.

The impact of childbirth on a woman's body is substantial, emphasizing the need for new mothers to focus keenly on their physical recovery. Every delivery, irrespective of the method, brings about significant changes and challenges that require time and proper attention to heal fully.

Childbirth is an intense physical endeavor, and it's common for new mothers to experience exhaustion, especially if sleep was elusive during the hospital stay. The weeks following the arrival of your baby are crucial for recovery. It's essential to use this time to rest whenever you can. Maximizing sleep during your baby's nap times is a practical way to help your body recover.

During this period, it's also important to set boundaries regarding visitors. You're not obligated to entertain guests, and it's perfectly acceptable to prioritize your rest and recovery. If you need to, feel free to excuse yourself for a nap or to care for your baby. This time is about your health and adjusting to your new role as a mother, so taking care of yourself should be your top priority.

If you've had a cesarean section, it's particularly important to manage your physical activity during the recovery period. Doctors commonly advise avoiding lifting anything heavier than your baby to prevent straining your healing incision. Rest is crucial, not just for recovery from the surgery but also for coping with the demands of a new baby.

Nourishment plays a vital role in your recovery process. The weight gained during pregnancy isn't just extra pounds; it serves as vital energy reserves that support both recovery and breastfeeding. Lactation experts recommend that breastfeeding mothers should eat according to their hunger but also focus on the quality and balance of their meals. It's essential to ensure that your diet includes a variety of foods such as fruits, vegetables, grains, dairy products, and proteins. This helps in providing the necessary nutrients for both mother and child and aids in quicker recovery.

In the busy and often tiring routine with a newborn, it's easy to overlook your meal planning. Mothers might find themselves skipping meals due to fatigue or the demands of baby care. However, it's important to plan your meals. Prepare simple, nutritious meals that can be easily assembled. Keeping snacks like chopped vegetables, nuts, and fruit handy can also help maintain your energy levels throughout the day. Taking these steps ensures that you do not neglect your dietary needs, which is crucial for your recovery and well-being as a new mother.

After childbirth, mothers begin on a complex journey, navigating physical recovery and emotional changes. It's crucial to be aware of specific warning signs that require immediate medical attention to ensure the health and well-being of both the mother and the baby.

Postpartum Depression and Baby Blues: Postpartum depression is a severe condition that can affect any new mother, regardless of how her baby was delivered. Feeling slightly disconnected or down during the first week after childbirth is common; this is often referred to as the "baby blues." However, if these feelings persist beyond two weeks or if the mother experiences overwhelming sadness, anxiety, or thoughts of harming herself or the baby, it is critical to seek professional help immediately.

Physical Changes and Recovery: After giving birth, most mothers will experience a vaginal discharge known as lochia. This discharge is heavy and red at first, resembling a menstrual period, but it gradually lightens to pink and then to a pale white or yellow color over the weeks following delivery. It's essential for mothers to monitor the discharge and consult healthcare providers if there are any concerns, such as an unusually heavy flow or a foul smell, which could indicate an infection.

Pelvic Floor Health: Many women experience stress incontinence due to the stretching or injury of pelvic floor muscles during delivery. Factors such as obesity, multiple pregnancies, prolonged breastfeeding, smoking, or the use of forceps can increase the risk of urinary incontinence shortly after childbirth. Engaging in pelvic floor exercises and seeking advice from healthcare professionals can help manage and mitigate these issues.

Sexual Health and Intimacy: It's not uncommon for women to have a diminished interest in sexual activity after childbirth, primarily due to hormonal changes. Estrogen levels may take up to a year to return to pre-pregnancy levels. Additionally, physical discomfort, fatigue, and concerns about pregnancy can affect sexual desire. Open communication with your partner about these changes can help both partners adjust and understand each other's needs during this time.

Breastfeeding Challenges: Breastfeeding, while beneficial for both mother and baby, can come with its set of challenges, such as difficulties with latching or inadequate milk supply. Seeking support and guidance from lactation consultants can provide essential help, ensuring that both the mother and baby are comfortable and well-nourished.

Navigating the postpartum period involves monitoring these aspects closely and communicating openly with healthcare providers about any concerns. Understanding these common issues can significantly reduce stress and enhance the experience of caring for a new baby. Remember, it's always better to discuss any small concerns with your doctor than to wait until they become more significant problems. Taking proactive steps towards addressing these issues not only ensures your health but also helps you enjoy your journey into motherhood with more confidence and less anxiety.

Reflecting on Growth

Pregnancy is a profound period of transformation that extends beyond physical changes, marking a significant phase of personal growth and transition into parenthood. As you navigate through each trimester, your body undergoes remarkable changes that prepare you not just for childbirth but for the lifelong journey of parenting.

This period offers a unique opportunity to reflect on your growth, as you learn to adapt to the evolving needs of your body and the little life developing inside you. It's a time when many expectant mothers begin to connect deeply with their inner strength, resilience, and capacity for nurturing.

The physical growth during pregnancy is visible and often celebrated, but the emotional and psychological growth is equally significant. Embracing this growth involves acknowledging the fears and uncertainties that come with impending motherhood while also celebrating the joys and anticipations of meeting your child. It's a transformative experience that reshapes your identity, priorities, and perspectives.

Understanding and accepting these changes can be empowering. It encourages a positive outlook towards labor and delivery, which are not just the culmination of pregnancy but also the beginning of a new chapter in life. The journey through pregnancy to parenthood is an extraordinary passage that prepares you for the demands and delights of raising a child. This reflection on growth helps build a foundation of awareness and adaptability, essential for the challenges and rewards that lie ahead in parenting.

Accepting Change

Adapting to the changes that come with pregnancy is essential for preparing for the challenges of parenthood. Pregnancy brings a host of changes—physical, emotional, and psychological. Here are effective strategies to help manage these transitions:

Learn as Much as Possible: Knowledge about what happens during each trimester can reduce anxiety and stress. Participate in prenatal classes, read relevant literature, and engage in discussions on platforms dedicated to pregnancy and parenting.

Keep Communication Open: Maintaining open dialogue with your partner, family, and healthcare provider is crucial. Sharing your feelings and experiences can garner support and understanding. It's important to vocalize your needs and emotions.

Prioritize Your Health: A healthy lifestyle during pregnancy is vital. Focus on eating well-balanced meals, performing pregnancy-safe exercises, and securing adequate rest. These habits are pivotal for your overall well-being and the health of your baby.

Plan for the Future: Anticipate the changes that a new baby will bring. Discuss with your partner how you plan to manage different aspects of parenting. Arranging for help after the baby arrives can also mitigate stress during the transition into parenthood.

Accept Changes: Understanding that change is a part of the journey can help you mentally prepare for the impact of pregnancy. Accepting these changes can give resilience and adaptability, which are valuable in parenthood.

The First Steps

Entering parenthood is a transformative journey filled with new experiences and adjustments. It's a time when every day can bring something new, as you and your baby start to get to know each other. Here's a closer look at what you might expect in the early stages of this adventure.

From the moment you bring your newborn home, life changes. Your old routines might no longer fit as you now operate on a schedule that meets the needs of your baby. This can include frequent feedings—day and night—changing diapers, and soothing sessions, which can all feel overwhelming at first. However, these moments are also opportunities to bond deeply with your new child, learning each other's cues and developing a unique rhythm together.

Emotionally, it's natural to feel a mix of joy, fear, excitement, and sometimes anxiety. These feelings are compounded by significant hormonal changes occurring in your body after childbirth. It's important to allow yourself to fully experience these emotions and share them with your partner or a supportive friend or family member. Open communication can help ease the emotional load of early parenthood.

Bonding with your baby is one of the most fulfilling aspects of early parenting. Simple actions like holding your baby close, making eye contact, and talking softly help to strengthen your connection. These interactions not only comfort your baby but also promote emotional and physical well-being for both of you.

Interpreting your baby's needs initially might seem like a mystery. With time, you'll start to recognize what different cries might mean and what can soothe your baby most effectively. Trust in your growing parental instincts and remember that it's perfectly fine to seek advice from those with more experience or from your pediatrician.

Ensuring your baby's health includes regular pediatric check-ups. These visits are crucial for monitoring your baby's development and getting professional guidance. Use these appointments to voice any concerns and learn from the healthcare professionals who are there to support your parenting journey.

Remember that you also need support. Building a network of friends, and family, or joining parenting groups can provide emotional solace and practical help. Parenting is often more manageable and enjoyable when you have others to share the experiences with.

Do not neglect your own well-being. Caring for yourself by eating nutritious foods, resting when possible, and finding time for personal relaxation is essential. The better you feel, the more you will enjoy this special time with your new baby.

Each day as a new parent may bring challenges, but it also brings immense joy and satisfaction.

Watching your baby grow and respond to their development with love and attention is one of the most rewarding aspects of life. Embrace this time with all its ups and downs, as these early days are precious steps on the wonderful journey of parenthood.

*"Birth is not only about making babies.
Birth is about making mothers—strong,
competent, capable mothers who trust
themselves and know their inner strength."
– Barbara Katz Rothman*

Action Item

Spend quality time with your partner discussing your hopes and fears about parenthood. Consider writing a letter to your future child about your hopes and dreams for them.

Conclusion

It's a moment to reflect on the journey that leads to parenthood. This experience, filled with anticipation, learning, and personal growth, reshapes our lives in unimaginable ways. It's a journey that stretches the limits of our emotions and endurance, enriching our world with a new depth of love and responsibility.

Celebrating this journey means recognizing the strength it took to accept the changes that came with each trimester, the courage to face the uncertainties of delivery, and the resilience to adapt to life with a new baby. It's about appreciating the small victories—each doctor's visit that went well, the successful completion of a nursery, or the support we found in our partners and loved ones.

Transitioning to parenthood is not just about the birth of a child; it's the birth of new parents. This role, brimming with challenges and rewards, is one of life's most significant transformations. As we step into this role, it's essential to carry forward the gratitude for the journey that's shaped us—acknowledging the support systems that held us up, the medical care that guided us safely, and the personal growth that readied us for the days ahead.

Reflecting on these experiences with gratitude allows us to embrace parenthood with a renewed sense of purpose and optimism. It prepares us to give our children the love, security, and nurturing they need to thrive. As new chapters in life await, we move forward enriched by our experiences, ready to teach, learn, and grow alongside our children in the incredible adventure of parenting.

Additional Chapter: Case Studies

Life is full of miracles. No one can predict the future, but as an obstetrician, I've learned that we can often anticipate the likelihood of certain outcomes based on experience. Throughout my career, I have encountered cases that seemed touched by an invisible force, moments when an unseen energy appeared to guide us through the extraordinary challenges and joys of childbirth. Here, I share some of these remarkable experiences—each one a reminder of the mysterious and powerful forces at play in the journey of bringing new life into the world.

Case Study 1

In the first case, we encountered a Muslim patient who was notably obese, weighing around 98 kilograms and was experiencing labor pains. She had diligently attended all her regular antenatal visits with a couple of doctors in her area. During her examination, it was discovered that the baby was positioned in a breech; this means the baby's head was up, and the buttocks were pointed down towards the birth canal. I discussed with her and her family the significant risks associated with delivering a breech baby vaginally, especially given the baby's substantial weight of more than 3.5 kilograms and the complication of the umbilical cord being wrapped around the baby's neck.

Despite the risks, the family decided to proceed with a vaginal delivery after understanding all the potential outcomes. We prepared for the possibility of needing an emergency cesarean section, alerting the necessary medical staff and ensuring all consent forms were signed and understood. Remarkably, the delivery was successful, and the mother was able to give birth vaginally to a healthy baby weighing over 3.5 kilograms without any complications.

Conversely, another patient of mine was in a different yet challenging situation. She was anticipating her second child, and her first child had been delivered normally two years earlier. However, during this pregnancy, the baby was again in a breech position but with additional complications including a deflexed head and a tightly wrapped umbilical cord. Despite the clear risks to the baby's well-being during a normal vaginal delivery, the family was hesitant to opt for a cesarean section. With their informed consent, we proceeded with a trial of labor, hoping for a normal delivery. Unfortunately, during the delivery, the baby's head became stuck at the pelvic brim due to its awkward positioning, and the baby did not cry immediately after birth, despite efforts at resuscitation.

In managing breech deliveries, we utilize a breech scoring index that helps us predict the complexity of the delivery early on, often right at admission, provided the labor has been active prior. This scoring system is crucial as it helps identify both overt and subtler cases of fetopelvic disproportion through a numerical value ranging from 0 to 3, with lower scores indicating a higher likelihood of complications.

A score of 4 on this scale suggests potential issues, warranting further assessments, often including radiological evaluations, to determine the safest course of action. If the score is high, it typically means the breech delivery should proceed without significant problems. In situations where labor is abnormal, we might use oxytocic drugs to facilitate the process effectively.

It's important to understand that this breach score is a tool to assist in clinical decision-making—it doesn't replace the expertise and judgment of an experienced obstetrician. Instead, it visually summarizes the various factors an obstetrician must consider, helping guide whether to continue with a vaginal delivery in a breech presentation or opt for a cesarean section. This approach is part of our commitment to ensuring the best outcomes for mother and baby, relying on sound medical judgment and the latest in diagnostic tools.

These cases show how important it is to trust your doctor. As in any profession, the advice of a specialist, in this case, an obstetrician, is based on years of training and experience focused on the best outcomes for both mother and child. Doctors are trained to assess and manage the risks associated with different types of deliveries. They aim to ensure the best possible outcomes for both mother and baby. I encourage all expectant parents to trust their doctors' advice. It's important to allow your healthcare team to make the best decisions based on their expertise and understanding of your specific medical situation. Remember, they are equipped with the knowledge and experience to navigate complex delivery scenarios safely.

"A baby is God's opinion that the
world should go on."
– Carl Sandburg

Case Study 2

The approach to childbirth after a cesarean section has shifted significantly, now offering the option of vaginal birth after cesarean (VBAC) as a viable and safe alternative for many women. This change in guidelines, supported by the American Congress of Obstetricians and Gynecologists (ACOG), reflects a broader acceptance of VBAC for women who have had one or two previous cesarean deliveries.

When considering VBAC, it is crucial to consult with your healthcare provider to determine the best course of action based on your individual health and the specifics of your previous deliveries. Although VBAC carries benefits, it also presents risks such as uterine rupture or severe bleeding. These complications necessitate delivering in a well-equipped facility under the care of experienced medical professionals.

Consider the story of a patient from a lower economic background who arrived in the labor room with intense contractions. Despite having undergone two cesarean sections previously, the urgent nature of her situation led to a rapid decision-making process without the usual formalities of consent. Fortunately, she delivered a healthy baby shortly thereafter. This case highlights the unpredictable nature of childbirth and the importance of expert care during such critical moments.

The Benefits of VBAC?

Opting for a Vaginal Birth After Cesarean (VBAC) can offer several substantial benefits, enhancing the overall birth experience and potentially leading to better outcomes in subsequent pregnancies. According to the Mayo Clinic, the advantages of choosing a VBAC include:

- **Quicker Recovery:** Women who deliver vaginally generally experience shorter hospital stays. This not only reduces medical costs but also allows for a faster return to normal activities.

- **Increased Participation:** Experiencing a vaginal birth can provide a more profound sense of involvement in the birthing process. Many women report feeling more connected to the experience, which can be empowering.

- **Reduced Risks in Future Pregnancies:** Choosing VBAC can decrease the risks associated with multiple cesarean sections, such as infections, organ damage, and excessive blood loss. For those planning to have more children, VBAC might be the safer option to minimize complications in future deliveries.

The National Institutes of Health (NIH) supports these benefits, noting that a successful VBAC is often the safest method for a woman who has previously undergone a cesarean delivery. Statistics show that the success rate for women who attempt a trial of labor for VBAC is between 60 and 80 percent. This successful transition reduces the necessity for surgical intervention, aligning with efforts to promote natural birth processes whenever safely possible.

While a Vaginal Birth After Cesarean (VBAC) offers many benefits, it's not without its risks, one of the most severe being the possibility of uterine rupture. Uterine rupture occurs when the uterus tears along the scar line from a previous cesarean delivery. This complication can be life-threatening and usually requires an emergency cesarean delivery to prevent serious outcomes such as heavy bleeding and infection in the mother, and potential brain damage in the baby.

In some severe cases, a hysterectomy, which involves the removal of the uterus, may be necessary after a uterine rupture. This procedure would prevent any future pregnancies, which is a significant consideration for women planning larger families. Despite these concerns, the American Congress of Obstetricians and Gynecologists (ACOG) reports that the risk of uterine rupture for women who have had a low transverse incision in a previous cesarean is relatively low, about 1 in 500. This statistic suggests that while the risk is real, it is infrequent, allowing many women to safely consider VBAC under the right medical guidance.

Determining if you are a good candidate for a Vaginal Birth After Cesarean (VBAC) involves considering several factors that can influence the likelihood of a successful vaginal delivery. These factors include:

- **Fetal Position:** The optimal position for a successful VBAC is when the baby is head down.

- **Baby's Size:** Ideally, the baby should weigh less than 3 kilograms (about 7 pounds, 11 ounces) to increase the chances of a successful VBAC.

- **Previous Vaginal Delivery:** Having had a successful vaginal delivery in the past can significantly improve your chances of a successful VBAC, sometimes by more than 90%.

- **Reason for Previous Cesarean:** If the reason for your previous cesarean is not a factor in this pregnancy, it may increase your chances of having a successful VBAC.

- **Type of Uterine Incision:** A low transverse incision is preferable for VBAC. A vertical or T-shaped scar may increase the risk of complications.

- **Natural Labor Onset:** Spontaneous labor is ideal. Induction can increase the risk of uterine rupture due to stronger and faster contractions.

However, the likelihood of a successful VBAC decreases if:

- You go past your due date.

- You have had more than two previous cesarean deliveries.

Certain conditions make VBAC unsafe, such as a history of uterine rupture or a vertical incision from a previous cesarean.

To prepare for a possible VBAC:

- Discuss extensively with your doctor to understand your chances based on your medical history and current pregnancy condition.

- Choose a healthcare provider and hospital that are experienced and supportive of VBACs and equipped for emergency situations.

- Consider taking a childbirth class that covers VBAC to educate yourself and your partner about the process and expectations.

- Plan for natural labor onset, if possible, as induction can increase risks.

- Prepare mentally for any outcome, including the possibility of another cesarean section if complications arise during labor.

The decision should focus on what is safest for both you and your baby, with the goal being a healthy delivery regardless of the method.

- **Review Your Medical History:** Your doctor will review your medical records from previous pregnancies to identify any recurring issues or potential complications that could affect a VBAC.

- **Assess Current Pregnancy:** Evaluate your current pregnancy's progress with your doctor. This includes checking the baby's position, your health, and other pregnancy-related factors that could influence delivery methods.

- **Make an Informed Decision:** Using the information from your discussions and evaluations, you and your doctor can make an informed decision about whether to attempt a VBAC or opt for a repeat cesarean delivery.

- **Plan for Both Scenarios:** Prepare for both potential outcomes. Even if you and your doctor decide to try for a VBAC, it's essential to understand that circumstances could change, and a cesarean might become necessary.

Ultimately, the goal is to ensure the safety and health of both you and your baby. Making an informed decision with your doctor based on your medical history and current pregnancy conditions will help you achieve the best outcome.

"A mother's love for her child is like nothing else in the world. It knows no law, no pity, it dates all things and crushes down remorselessly all that stands in its path."
– Agatha Christie

Case Study 3

In this particular case, a woman who had previously had a C-section came into the labor room with strong contractions and a lot of labor pain. During her check-up, doctors found that the baby weighed 3.9 kg and she was fully ready for delivery—the cervix was completely open and everything was in place for the baby to come out. Amazingly, just 10 to 15 minutes later, she gave birth to a healthy baby without any complications.

This story really shows that even if a mother has had a C-section before, she can still have a natural birth the next time if everything lines up right. It's important for moms to stay open to all possibilities—natural or C-section—because you never know what will happen when the time comes. It also shows how crucial it is for doctors to be ready for anything. They need to be quick to make decisions and skilled in both types of deliveries to ensure the best care for both mom and baby.

> *"Life doesn't come with a manual,*
> *it comes with a mother."*
> *– Unknown*

Case Study 4

Emergency situations in childbirth often lead to difficult decisions that must be made quickly to ensure the safety of both mother and baby. This was the case during a particularly challenging delivery situation that occurred shortly after a patient was admitted to the hospital. The patient, who had previously had a cesarean section, began to experience strong labor pains and contractions, indicating that the baby might soon be delivered.

As the labor progressed, the medical team closely monitored the mother's vital signs, such as blood pressure and heart rate, as well as the baby's heart rate. Every few hours, the doctors checked how the baby was positioned and how far the labor had advanced. Despite these efforts, the baby's progress was slower than expected. When it became clear that the baby's head was not moving down into the birth canal as it should, the doctors prepared for the possibility of another cesarean section.

However, the situation took a turn when the anesthetist was delayed due to unforeseen circumstances, causing a 45-minute wait. During this time, the mother's contractions grew stronger. Upon re-examining the mother, the doctors saw a new opportunity for a vaginal delivery using a vacuum extraction method. Despite the initial plan for a cesarean and the relatives' concerns about the risks, the medical team decided to proceed with the vacuum delivery.

Fortunately, the decision proved successful. The baby was delivered safely and began crying immediately after birth, indicating good health. This case explains the unpredictable nature of childbirth and the importance of flexibility and quick thinking in medical decision-making. It also highlights the critical role of trust between patients, their families, and medical professionals during such tense moments.

> *"A mother's love is patient and forgiving*
> *when all others are forsaking, it never*
> *fails or falters, even though the*
> *heart is breaking."*
> *– Helen Rice*

Case Study 5

In this particular instance, a patient arrived at our hospital after enduring an extended and challenging labor, having been transferred from a remote location. During the initial examination, it was discovered that the fetal head was deeply impacted in the pelvis, showing signs of caput and moulding. Tragically, there was no detectable heartbeat, indicating that the baby had not survived.

Despite the initial recommendation for a cesarean section due to these complications, the expertise of our medical team led to a different course of action. They opted for a less common, but in this case, appropriate procedure known as a destructive delivery. This allowed the delivery to proceed normally, avoiding the need for a cesarean section.

This decision significantly reduced the hospital stay and minimized the mother's postpartum recovery issues. This case underscores the critical role of skilled healthcare providers in making informed, sensitive decisions that prioritize the mother's health and well-being in complex obstetric scenarios.

*"The only creatures that are evolved
enough to convey pure love are
dogs and infants."*
– Johnny Depp

Case Study 6

In this case, we explore the journey of a mother who conceived through in vitro fertilization (IVF) and was committed to a natural delivery, despite recommendations for a cesarean section. Throughout her pregnancy, she engaged actively in prenatal classes and followed all recommended antenatal care routines, fostering a strong belief in her ability to deliver naturally.

When labor began, she presented with effective, natural labor pains. Initial examinations showed that her cervix was dilated to 3 to 4 cm, and the baby was in a good position without any complications like caput or molding. However, during delivery, she encountered a challenging situation with shoulder dystocia, a condition where the baby's shoulders have difficulty passing through the birth canal.

Thanks to the swift and skilled response of the medical team, the baby was delivered safely through specialized maneuvers for managing shoulder dystocia. Immediately after birth, though the baby cried well, a complication arose—accidental pneumothorax, a condition where air leaks into the space between the lung and chest wall. The newborn required intensive care, spending 15 to 20 days in the ICU.

Despite these challenges, the mother's positive attitude and hope played a crucial role in their journey. Ultimately, the baby recovered well and was joyfully reunited with the mother. This case highlights the unpredictable nature of childbirth and the importance of preparedness and resilience in the face of unexpected challenges.

> *"Children reinvent your world for you."*
> *– Susan Sarandon*

Case Study 7

In this case, we explore a common concern during childbirth: the presence of a cord around the baby's neck. While the idea of a nuchal cord (cord around the neck) can cause significant anxiety for families, it's important to understand that it isn't always a direct indication for a cesarean section. With careful intrapartum monitoring, many babies with nuchal cords—including those with multiple loops—can be safely delivered vaginally.

The key is vigilant monitoring during labor to detect any signs of fetal distress, such as changes in the baby's heart rate or the presence of meconium-stained amniotic fluid, which can indicate that the baby has experienced stress. In cases where fetal distress is confirmed, transitioning to a cesarean delivery might become necessary to ensure the safety of both mother and baby.

One notable instance from my practice involved a baby with four loops of the cord around the neck. We prepared for an emergency cesarean section, ensuring all necessary precautions and equipment were ready in the operating room. Remarkably, the baby was delivered vaginally without any complications, resulting in a healthy male child. This patient later went on to have a vaginal breech delivery and a third vaginal delivery of a baby with intrauterine growth restriction (IUGR), reinforcing the principle that a successful first vaginal delivery can set a positive precedent for future deliveries.

This case illustrates the importance of skilled obstetric care and the need to evaluate each situation individually. It highlights that while a nuchal cord can present challenges, with the right conditions and expert monitoring, successful vaginal delivery is very possible.

Conclusion

Each story serves as a testament to the complexity and unpredictability of childbirth. They underscore the importance of skilled medical guidance and the need for adaptability in managing each unique situation. Whether it involves an emergency cesarean section, a successful vaginal birth after cesarean (VBAC), or navigating the challenges of a nuchal cord, these cases highlight the critical role of informed decision-making and trust between healthcare providers and patients.

This also reminds us of the miraculous nature of birth and the resilience of both mothers and medical teams. They celebrate the victories of childbirth, where careful monitoring and expert care can lead to outcomes that defy the odds, bringing new life into the world safely and joyfully. Through these stories, we gain a deeper appreciation for the art and science of obstetrics, and the profound impact of having a supportive, knowledgeable team during one of life's most significant moments.